Living...Without Milk

Living...Without Milk

A cookbook and nutritional guide for
those who should avoid dairy products

by

Jacqueline Hostage

Illustrations by Robin Hostage Toth

Cover design by Edward G. Foss

Betterway Publications
White Hall, Virginia

Third edition

First Printing: April, 1981

Published by Betterway Publications
White Hall, Virginia 22987

Copyright © 1981 by Jacqueline Hostage
All rights reserved. No part of this book may be reproduced, by any means, except by a reviewer who wishes to quote brief excerpts in connection with a review in a magazine or newspaper.

Library of Congress Cataloging in Publication Data
Hostage, Jacqueline E.
   Living--without milk.

   Includes index.
  1. Milk-free diet--Recipes. 1. Title.

RM234.5H67 1981	641.5′63	81-1271
ISBN 0-932620-06-X	(Library Edition)	AACR2
ISBN 0-932620-05-1	(Paper Edition)	

Printed in the United States of America

This book is lovingly dedicated to Joshua and Sarah. Of course, every grandmother thinks her grandchildren are the best and the brightest. Mine really are.

FOREWORD

In theory, milk is a nutritious food. In fact, the human body often may not metabolize milk well - in any of its forms. This inability, evidenced in individuals who are allergic to milk or who are lactose intolerant, may cause physical and emotional disorders that often are difficult to diagnose.

For several years, I have been "prescribing" an earlier edition of **Living...Without Milk** to patients of mine who need help in managing their milk-free diets. When the author asked me to prepare a chapter for this new edition, fully defining lactose intolerance, I was pleased to do so.

Whether your reason for requiring a milk-free diet is lactose intolerance or milk allergy, this updated and expanded nutritional guide and cookbook should be of great benefit.

                Lee Sataline, M.D., F.A.C.P., AGA, ASGE
                Internist and Gastroenterologist

CONTENTS

PART ONE: An introduction to milk related health problems

Milk: Not a "Natural" for Millions 11
Lactose Intolerance by Dr. Lee Sataline.................. 15
The Milk-free Diet: Foods to Avoid 18
Products to Check Carefully 20
Pull-out Diet Chart 23
A Word About Nutrition............................... 25
Making Milk Easier to Digest 29
Tofu: The Versatile Soy Cheese 31
Special Help for Milk-free Diets 35

PART TWO: Delicious, nutritious milk-free recipes for every occasion

Super Substitutes for Convenience Foods 37
Milk free alternatives to packaged foods
Standard Recipes You Still Can Use..................... 47
Making the most of your cookbooks
New Beginnings: The Better Breakfast.................. 49
    Omelets   Pancakes   Muffins
    Coffee Cakes   Breakfast Cookies
    Meals-in-a-Glass
Appetizers & Dips..................................... 57
Breaking the "cheese and crackers" routine
Main Dishes.. 63
    Meat   Poultry   Seafood
    Eggs   Meat Alternatives
Accompaniments 81
    Vegetables   Rice   Noodles
Soups & Salads 89
    Speedy Soups   Super Salads
Baked Goods 99
    Breads   Biscuits   Cookies
    Cakes   Pies   Pastries
Happy Endings....................................... 119
    Refrigerator and Frozen Desserts
    Confections   Ice Cream

PART THREE: Where to go for more information

Product Information Directory 127
Other Sources of Help 131

General Index 132
Recipe Index 134

MILK: NOT A "NATURAL" FOR MILLIONS

Some of the most commonly consumed foods - milk and milk products - are the underlying causes of many physical and emotional illnesses. Although milk is a product with which most of us have grown up, accepting it as an essential part of our diet, it can cause a variety of symptoms in many of us that frequently are misdiagnosed or untreated. The medical literature covering symptoms attributed to milk allergy or intolerance involves a cross-section of the population: young and old; those who rarely ever drink milk and those who are heavy milk drinkers; people of every ethnic and economic background. Authorities have estimated that 30 million Americans and most of the rest of the world's adult population suffer from a condition called "lactose intolerance". Almost as many people are plagued by an allergy to milk.

While lactose intolerance and milk allergy are the most common problems attributed to milk, the case against milk consumption is strengthened by studies in other fields, as well. Both Dr. K. Oster, chief cardiology emeritus at Park City Hospital in Bridgeport, Connecticut and Dr. J. Annand have conducted studies that relate heated milk (particularly the homogenized variety) to forms of heart disease. Dr. Oster assigns the blame to an enzyme in cow's milk called xanthine oxidase which causes problems by attacking the heart's arteries.

Although milk is not the villain in every case, researchers and physicians have demonstrated that allergic reactions or sensitivities frequently mimic or even *cause* a host of symptoms - symptoms that frustrate and affect diagnosis. Some of these include: abdominal swelling, arthritis, asthma, canker sores, chronic cough, colitis, constipation, depression, diarrhea, ear infections, eczema, fatigue, hyperactivity, iron deficiency anemia, psychosis, ulcers, and even hidden bleeding in infants from injuries to the intestinal tract.

The all-too-common result of failing to recognize the role that milk allergy or sensitivity may play is the misdiagnosis and treatment of the problem. Let's look at some cases where individuals were helped by recognition of the fact the "real" problem was the inability to metabolize milk properly.

In his book, *5-Day Allergy Relief System,* Dr. Marshall Mandell cites many cases of chronic illnesses that are based on allergic reactions to milk. He has found, for example, that a few drops of milk could induce a state of deep depresson in a sensitive patient. One 16-year old schizophrenic was relieved of her symptoms by a four day fast, but became psychotic again after a glass of milk. A forty-eight year old woman relived all the pain of a perforated ulcer (removed one month earlier) upon being administered a sublingual (under the tongue) test for milk sensitivity. A patient, who had been treated for colitis for eight years, found her condition eliminated after Dr. Mandell supervised a therapeutic milk-free fast for her. Another case involved a man who suffered extreme fatigue after his frequently enjoyed lunchtime milk and ice cream.

Dr. Mandell is not alone in demonstrating that allergic reactions in the brain and other parts of the nervous system can be provoked by allergic reactions to food in general and milk - one of the most allergenic foods in America - in particular. Dr. W.H. Philpott reports in his book, *Brain Allergies,* that fifty-one percent of the 250 consecutive, unselected emotionally disturbed patients treated in his own practice exhibited symptoms when exposed to pasteurized whole milk.

Dr. Theron Randolph, who did some of the earlier work that led Dr. Mandell to pursue the connection between milk allergy and ulcers, was also successful in treating rheumatoid arthritis in his allergy patients - many of whom were allergic to milk. Dr. A.H. Rowe, Dr. J.A. Trumbull, and others have contributed clinical evidence supporting the conclusion that the principal cause of rheumatoid arthritis in many cases is simple allergy to food.

Perhaps even more common than allergy to milk is sensitivity to milk, or lactose intolerance. When a test group of children who suffered recurrent stomach aches were studied by Dr. Melvin Levine at Harvard Medical School, forty percent were found to be lactose intolerant. Removing milk from their diets ended their problems and precluded the series of x-rays and tests to which they otherwise unecessarily might been exposed.

As the above has indicated, some individuals have a true allergy to milk and react to it in any form. Others are milk intolerant; that is, their systems lack the enzyme (lactase) necessary to digest the milk sugar (lactose) in milk. How do you find out if milk is *your* problem? Your doctor, by performing certain laboratory tests, can usually determine the cause of your allergy or whether or not you are lactose intolerant.

In the case of an allergy, the most common method used is to keep a careful record of all foods eaten along with the notation of any symptoms of allergy. This, followed by the elimination of milk and milk products from the diet and the subsequent relief of the symptoms, may identify an allergy to milk. (Skin tests are less likely to be used in determining food allergy than they are in determining contact allergies because of their questionable reliability.) Some allergists use the sublingual technique which involves placing dilutions of food extracts under the tongue.

The determination of lactose (milk sugar) intolerance is complicated by the fact that many individuals can tolerate *some* milk in their diet. As a result, symptoms do not always show up immediately (as they are more likely to do with an allergy). With lactose intolerance, Monday's cheese sandwich may not trigger an attack of diarrhea until Friday. However, a determination of milk sugar sensitivity can be made through the use of a simple and reliable blood test which measures the blood sugar level at fasting and again at various intervals (over a period of several hours after ingesting flavored lactose). Another method, the breath-hydrogen test, involves ingestion of a heavy "load" of lactose followed by the analysis of breath samples (taken periodically over a two-hour period) for hydrogen content. Either test may be preceded or followed by trial diets (both lactose-containing and lactose-free) combined with careful record keeping.

What are your chances of having either problem? An accumulation of medical and scientific research evidence confirms that lactose intolerance and milk allergies run in families. Even if only one parent has either or bother problems, the likelihood is that one or more of the family's children will inherit one or both conditions. In addition, since the lactase enzyme commonly disappears or diminishes during the aging process, older adults frequently develop lactose intolerance in later years. Since the symptoms that develop may represent an organic or emotional disease, each case requires careful evaluation by a physician.

Faced with a confirmed diagnosis of either problem, your best defense is a cautious approach to food selection and preparation. Become an avid label reader. Prepare as many meals from "scratch" as possible so you know exactly what ingredients you are serving - and eating. Avoiding milk is not difficult once you become familiar with all of its varied forms. While cheese, ice cream, butter, and yogurt readily come to mind as milk products, cow's milk contains lactose, whey, lactalbumin, casein, and dozens of other natural chemicals, some of which form the basis for additives that we find in other foods.

The purpose of this book is not only to help you prepare more interesting meals without the use of milk or milk products but to help you identify the "hidden" ingredients that contrbute to the problem. Additives used in this country total more than three pounds per person annually and the use of additives is increasing. For example, mono-sodium-glutamate, now manufactured from wheat, corn, and sugar-beet by-products, is an ingredient in more than 10,000 processed foods. Many food product labels do not even mention its presence.

Your doctor can help you decide which foods and additives you should avoid after he has determined the nature and extent of your problem. Knowing exactly what is in everything you eat will be a challenge initially but take comfort from the fact that it becomes easier as you familiarize yourself with the ingredients in your favorite products and as you prepare the dishes using only basic, milk-free ingredients.

LACTOSE INTOLERANCE

Irritable bowel syndrome, the most common gastrointestinal disorder seen by physicians, is characterized by a variety of complaints ranging from postprandial distress, bloating, pain, diarrhea and/or constipation, indigestion, etc. While most of these cases have been ascribed to psychogenic or emotional disorders it is not generally appreciated that lactose intolerance may be a major factor in the symptomatology.

Lactose intolerance has no prescribed set of symptoms. In some it may manifest itself solely by bloating and flatulence while in others there may be disturbances in bowel function ranging from diarrhea to abdominal cramping and constipation. It is impossible to ascribe the amount of lactose necessary to produce symptomatology in any one individual since it is difficult to ascertain the amount of lactose in an average American meal without purposely evaluating the content of the food stuffs involved. Frequently, patients and doctors will dismiss the diagnosis of lactose intolerance simply because the patient doesn't consume milk. These individuals do not realize that lactose is a common additive and filler to many American staples and since the intolerance is variable from one individual to the next no prescribed load of lactose can be incriminated. Furthermore, alcohol ingestion may reduce the tolerance. While milk allergy does exist, most children intolerant of milk suffer from lactose intolerance and are not truly allergic to milk.

It should be pointed out that lactose intolerance may be a primary disorder or secondary to some other intestinal disease, such as parasite infestation, inflammatory bowel disease or acute gastroenteritis due to a viral or bacterial agent. Often occult lactose intolerance is brought out by the acute onset of these acquired diseases. The patient in his desire to reduce the symptomatology of the infection will put himself on a "bland diet" containing large amounts of lactose, thereby aggravating the underlying disorder.

While lactose intolerance may involve any ethnic group it is very frequently found in the Black and Asian. However, the high incidence is also found in people whose ethnic background is of Mediterranean origin such as the Italians, Spanish, Lebanese, Jewish, etc. There is also a very high incidence of lactose intolerance in Polish and Slovak descendants. The American Indian has an extremely high incidence of lactose intolerance and it is incumbent on the physician to ascertain whether or not a patient has any Indian ancestry. This is common when dealing with French-Canadians and patients from the South or southwest United States. While the disorder is less common in patients of Anglo-Saxon or Nordic (Scandinavian) background, nevertheless, the incidence increases with age. Not infrequently there are elderly patients whose dyspeptic bowel symptoms are ascribed to "diverticulosis" when, in fact, they are lactose intolerant.

There are many idiosyncrasies and peculiarities

noted with lactose intolerance. A common and, as yet, unexplained phenomenon is the ability of a patient to drink chocolate milk while he cannot drink plain, white milk. Furthermore, it is not uncommon for patients to state that on one day they could consume with relative impunity a meal containing large amounts of lactose while the following day considerable distress occurred when the meal with even less lactose was consumed. No doubt some of this is due to the transit time of the lactose in the bowel yet many aspects of these phenomenon are not readily explainable. As the "sharpness" of the cheese is due to the fermentation of the lactose, a mild processed cheese is more apt to produce symptoms.

If I had one piece of advice to give all physicians treating gastrointestinal disorders I would say that irrespective of the symptoms any patient presenting with gastrointestinal complaints not associated with weight loss and who is not anemic or toxic should be screened for possible lactose intolerance. Considerable amounts of time, x-ray exposure and money would be saved if patients were first tested for this metabolic defect, rather than rushing them to the radiology departments. Colicky children with fecal incontinence and children with any type of abdominal complaint are more likely to have irritable bowel syndrome and/or lactose intolerance than any serious underlying gastrointestinal disorder. If this will only be remembered, the amount of radiation to which the children are exposed in the process of obtaining upper and lower gastrointestinal x-rays would be substantially reduced.

Lee Sataline, M.D., F.A.C.P., AGA, ASGE
Internist and Gastroenterologist

MILK-FREE DIET - FOODS TO AVOID

BEVERAGES: Made with milk or chocolate or cocoa preparations containing milk.

BAKED GOODS: All breads prepared with milk or milk products. Most commercial breads - except Kosher - contain milk or milk products. Soda crackers (check labels), doughnuts, popovers, pancakes, waffles, rusk, many crackers and cookies.

BREADED FOODS: Any containing milk or crumbs from bread, crackers, or cereal containing milk or milk products.

CEREALS: Any prepared with milk or containing milk or milk products. Check dry cereal package labels carefully.

DESSERTS: Cakes, cookies, puddings, or pie crusts made with milk. Bavarian creams, blanc-manges, custards, junket, ice cream, milk sherbet. Prepared mixes containing milk or milk products. Some commercial fruit fillings (check labels).

EGGS: Scrambled or creamed. Souffles.

FATS AND SALAD DRESSINGS: Butter, margarine made with milk or butter added. Salad dressings or boiled dressings containing milk, cream, butter, margarine, or cheese.

FRUITS: Canned or frozen prepared with lactose.

MEATS, POULTRY, FISH, SEAFOOD: Any prepared with milk or milk products. Many commercial dinners, hamburgers, frankfurters, sausages, and cold cuts - except Kosher - contain dry milk or other milk products.

MILK AND MILK PRODUCTS: Fresh, whole, and skim milk. Condensed, evaporated, dried milk, and milk solids. Cultured and buttermilk. Sweet or sour cream. Butter. All Cheeses. Powdered and malted milk. Powdered coffee creamer (check labels). Curds, wheys, casein*, sodium caseinate*, and lactalbumin*.

SAUCES AND GRAVIES: White, cream, butter or hard sauces or gravies made with milk or milk products or any prepared dish using these sauces.

SOUPS: Canned, homemade, or dried mixes containing milk or milk products.

VEGETABLES: Creamed or scalloped; potatoes that have been mashed with milk or cream.

MISCELLANEOUS: Creamed or scalloped foods; any dipped in milk or butter or fried in butter; any prepared with cheese. Any prepared mixes containing milk or milk products. Caramels, toffee, butterscotch, chocolate or any other candy containing milk or milk products.

DISCUSS WITH YOUR DOCTOR: Cocoa, chocolate, some instant coffee; chewing gum, powdered soft drinks, molasses, mono-sodium glutamate, party dips, blended spices, some dietetic and diabetic preparations. Cordials and liqueurs. Some medicines and vitamins. Sweetbreads, liver, brains. Corn, beets, peas, lima beans.

* These additives are from the protein of cow's milk and are permissible for those who cannot tolerate lactose (milk sugar) but not for those who are allergic to milk.

Living... Without Milk

PRODUCTS TO CHECK CAREFULLY

BREADS may contain milk, milk products, molasses or whey.

BREAD CRUMBS may contain the same ingredients as bread without being specifically identified on the label. In addition, they may contain mixed spices, cheese or mono-sodium-glutamate. The same cautions apply to CROUTONS.

CANDIES, especially filled candy bars, should be checked carefully.

COLD CUTS, FRANKFURTERS, AND SAUSAGES may contain milk or milk products.

COOKIES AND CRACKERS often contain milk, butter, whey, or lactose.

DELICATESSEN MEATS, such as roast beef or corned beef, may have been prepared using a tenderizer containing mono-sodium-glutamate.

FAST FOOD hamburgers, frankfurters, fried chicken, or fried fish may contain dried milk used as an extender or have milk in the batter.

FROZEN FOODS. Vegetables in sauces, hamburgers, T.V. dinners, baked goods - all may contain milk or milk products. Even fruit may be sweetened with lactose.

"KOSHER" FOODS are generally acceptable but watch for foods identified as "kosher" but with the additional word "dairy" which means that they contain dairy products (and under Jewish dietary laws can be eaten only with dairy meals). "Kosher" foods are usually identified by a "K" (alone or in a circle); with a "U" in a circle; or by a "P" or the word "Parve".

Products to Check Carefully

MAYONNAISE may contain mono-sodium-glutamate.

MIXED SPICES often contain lactose as a binder or mono-sodium-glutamate as a flavor enhancer.

MIXES OF ALL TYPES should be checked carefully - including: pudding and dessert mixes; bread, cake, and cookie mixes; rice mixes and seasoned coating mixes; and pancake, muffin, or biscuit mixes.

"NON-DAIRY" products such as powdered or liquid creamers and powered or frozen whipped toppings should all be checked carefully - some contain sodium caseinate, lactose, or whey solids.

PRESERVES AND JAMS occasionally have butter or margarine added to prevent the product from foaming during the manufacturing process.

RESTAURANTS are often heavy on the use of mono-sodium-glutamate, as well as butter and cream.

VITAMINS AND MEDICINES frequently use lactose as a binder. Often, this is not listed on the label so you should check with your doctor or write directly to the pharmaceutical company. If you are allergic to milk, avoid supplementing your diet with calcium lactate.

PHYSICIAN'S RECOMMENDATIONS AND NOTES

Pull-out Diet Chart

MILK-FREE DIET - FOODS TO AVOID

BEVERAGES: Made with milk or chocolate or cocoa preparations containing milk.

BAKED GOODS: All breads prepared with milk or milk products. Most commercial breads - except Kosher - contain milk or milk products. Soda crackers (check labels), doughnuts, popovers, pancakes, waffles, rusk, many crackers and cookies.

BREADED FOODS: Any containing milk or crumbs from bread, crackers, or cereal containing milk or milk products.

CEREALS: Any prepared with milk or containing milk or milk products. Check dry cereal package labels carefully.

DESSERTS: Cakes, cookies, puddings, or pie crusts made with milk. Bavarian creams, blancmanges, custards, junket, ice cream, milk sherbet. Prepared mixes containing milk or milk products. Some commercial fruit fillings (check labels).

EGGS: Scrambled or creamed. Souffles.

FATS AND SALAD DRESSINGS: Butter, margarine made with milk or butter added. Salad dressings or boiled dressings containing milk, cream, butter, margarine, or cheese.

FRUITS: Canned or frozen prepared with lactose.

MEATS, POULTRY, FISH, SEAFOOD: Any prepared with milk or milk products. Many commercial dinners, hamburgers, frankfurters, sausages, and cold cuts - except Kosher - contain dry milk or other milk products.

MILK AND MILK PRODUCTS: Fresh, whole, and skim milk. Condensed, evaporated, dried milk, and milk solids. Cultured and buttermilk. Sweet or sour cream. Butter. All Cheeses. Powdered and malted milk. Powdered coffee creamer (check labels). Curds, wheys, casein*, sodium caseinate*, and lactalbumin*.

SAUCES AND GRAVIES: White, cream, butter or hard sauces or gravies made with milk or milk products or any prepared dish using these sauces.

SOUPS: Canned, homemade, or dried mixes containing milk or milk products.

VEGETABLES: Creamed or scalloped; potatoes that have been mashed with milk or cream.

MISCELLANEOUS: Creamed or scalloped foods; any dipped in milk or butter or fried in butter; any prepared with cheese. Any prepared mixes containing milk or milk products. Caramels, toffee, butterscotch, chocolate or any other candy containing milk or milk products.

DISCUSS WITH YOUR DOCTOR: Cocoa, chocolate, some instant coffee; chewing gum, powdered soft drinks, molasses, monosodium-glutamate, party dips, blended spices, some dietetic and diabetic preparations. Cordials and liqueurs. Some medicines and vitamins. Sweetbreads, liver, brains. Corn, beets, peas, lima beans.

* These additives are from the protein of cow's milk and are permissible for those who cannot tolerate lactose (milk sugar) but not for those who are allergic to milk.

Living...Without Milk

PRODUCTS TO CHECK CAREFULLY

BREADS may contain milk, milk products, molasses or whey.

BREAD CRUMBS may contain the same ingredients as bread without being specifically identified on the label. In addition, they may contain mixed spices, cheese or mono-sodium-glutamate. The same cautions apply to CROUTONS.

CANDIES, especially filled candy bars, should be checked carefully.

COLD CUTS, FRANKFURTERS, AND SAUSAGES may contain milk or milk products.

COOKIES AND CRACKERS often contain milk, butter, whey, or lactose.

DELICATESSEN MEATS, such as roast beef or corned beef, may have been prepared using a tenderizer containing mono-sodium-glutamate.

FAST FOOD hamburgers, frankfurters, fried chicken, or fried fish may contain dried milk used as an extender or have milk in the batter.

FROZEN FOODS. Vegetables in sauces, hamburgers, t.v. dinners, baked goods - all may contain milk or milk products. Even fruit may be sweetened with lactose.

"KOSHER" FOODS are generally acceptable but watch for foods identified as "kosher" but with the additional word "dairy" which means that they contain dairy products (and under Jewish dietary laws can be eaten only with dairy meals). "Kosher" foods are usually identified by a "K" (alone or in a circle); with a "U" in a circle; or by a "P" or the word "Parve".

MAYONNAISE may contain mono-sodium-glutamate.

MIXED SPICES often contain mono-sodium-glutamate as a flavor enhancer.

MIXES OF ALL TYPES should be checked carefully - including: pudding and dessert mixes; bread, cake, and cookie mixes; rice mixes and seasoned coating mixes; and pancake, muffin, or biscuit mixes.

"NON-DAIRY" products such as powdered or liquid creamers and powdered or frozen whipped toppings should all be checked carefully - some contain sodium caseinate, lactose, or whey solids.

PRESERVES AND JAMS occasionally have butter or margarine added to prevent the product from foaming during the manufacturing process.

RESTAURANTS are often heavy on the use of mono-sodium-glutamate, as well as, butter and cream.

VITAMINS AND MEDICINES frequently use lactose as a binder. Often, this is not listed on the label so you should check with your doctor or write directly to the pharmaceutical company. If you are allergic to milk, avoid supplementing your diet with calcium lactate.

A WORD ABOUT NUTRITION

When eliminating a major food such as milk from the diet, thought must be given to the nutrients that also are being eliminated. A "lactose intolerant" is faced with a two-sided problem. First, because of your condition, you should not consume milk products, the source of so many valuable nutrients. However, if you do consume them anyway, you may be wasting the effort, because you may not digest or utilize them. Dr. David Paige, a pediatrician at John Hopkins University who has researched lactose intolerance, suggests that "people who don't digest milk well don't benefit from it nutritionally. And, if they don't, we should try to plan better diets using alternative foods for good nutrition".

We have prepared a chart (starting on page 27) which lists alternative food sources from which some of the nutrients found in milk products - protein, vitamin A, thiamin, riboflavin, and iron - may be obtained. Most American diets, through consumption of meats, poultry, fish, eggs, and beans, contain enough protein but other basic needs are more difficult to satisfy on a milk-free diet. Because of their special benefits, two additional nutrients are included on our chart.

The first is vitamin C. While some physicians deprecate the value of vitamin C, others feel that it plays a role in the management of allergies. In addition, investigators have found it dramatically boosts iron absorption when taken with meals. In fact, they indicate that the total intake of dietary iron is less critical than the availability of that iron to the system. Since iron is such an essential nutrient, the ability of vitamin C to help your system assimilate it could be important to you.

The second is potassium. While potassium is not one of the nutrients found primarily in milk, potassium deficiency often results from the chronic diarrhea frequently associated with lactose intolerance.

One look at the foods listed in the chart will illustrate why this cookbook contains so many recipes incorporating beans, bananas, and tofu. These ingredients offer so much value to the milk-free diet that we have tried to use as broad a sampling of recipes as possible. Consider the banana. Soft, bland, and easy to digest, it is often prescribed for the management of gastrointestinal disorders (including colitis, gastritis, and irritable colon), and its bulk is useful in the treatment of diarrhea. It is a readily available source of the potassium that is so important in maintaining the balance of body fluids and it provides a non-acidic source of vitamin C for ulcer patients. Finally, because of its hypoallergenic qualities, it is often used for patients with celiac disease or food allergies.

Notice that the figure in the last column of the chart shows the percentage of the U.S. Recommended Daily Allowance provided by a specific size portion of that food. Actually, not all people need 100% of the U.S. RDA for each nutrient every day. The U.S. Recommended Daily Allowances are the amounts used as standards in nutrition labeling; your personal needs are determined by your age, sex, and overall physical condition.

A young child, for example, may need only 80% of the U.S. RDA for calcium while a teenager or nursing mother may require 120%. The need for iron varies greatly, too, with women needing 100% until after menopause whereas 60% of the U.S. RDA will suffice for most adult males. An excellent reference for further information on individual nutritional requirements is the 57 page booklet, "Nutritional Labeling - tools for its use" (SN 001-000-03385-9) which is available for $1.15 from the Superintendent of Documents, U.S. Printing Office, Washington, DC 20402.

Follow your doctor's recommendations as to your individual requirements; then use the foods listed on the chart to help fulfill those needs. While supplements can serve a useful role, nutritionists have found that the vitamins found in food combine with the multiplicity of other nutritional factors in food for better absorption and utilization of all elements. Try to keep your diet as well balanced and varied as possible. And one more bit of counsel: since vitamin D is necessary for the absorption of calcium, be sure to take regular doses of sunshine!

NUTRIENTS: % U.S. RDA PROVIDED BY VARIOUS FOODS

NUTRIENT
Food and approximate measure — % U.S. RDA

VITAMIN A:
Food	% U.S. RDA
*Liver, beef, 3 ounces	910
Carrots, 1 cup diced, cooked	330
Spinach, 1 cup cooked	290
Sweet potato, 1 medium	180
Mixed vegetables, frozen, 1 cup cooked	180
Cantaloupe, half of 5-inch melon	180
Apricots, dried, cooked, 1 cup	150
Broccoli, 1 cup cooked	90
Prune juice, 1 cup	30
Asparagus, 1 cup cooked	25

THIAMIN (B1):
Food	% U.S. RDA
Pork chop, lean, 3 ounces	60
Sunflower seeds, ¼ cup	47
Ham, baked, 3 ounces	35
*Peas, 1 cup cooked	30
*Beans, dry (most varieties), 1 cup cooked	20
Asparagus, 1 cup cooked	15
Noodles or pasta, 1 cup cooked	15
Rice, 1 cup cooked	14
Avocado, cubed, 1 cup	10

RIBOFLAVIN (B2)
Food	% U.S. RDA
*Liver, beef, 3 ounces	210
Avocado, cubed, 1 cup	20
Mushrooms, raw, 1 cup	20
Broccoli, 1 cup cooked	17
Spinach, 1 cup cooked	15
Brussels sprouts, 1 cup cooked	15
Asparagus, 1 cup cooked	15

Living...Without Milk

NUTRIENT
Food and approximate measure % U.S. RDA

VITAMIN C:
Food	% U.S. RDA
Brussels sprouts, 1 cup cooked	230
Broccoli, 1 cup cooked	205
Pepper, raw, 1 medium	160
Cantaloupe, half of 5-inch melon	150
Strawberries, raw, 1 cup	150
Cauliflower, 1 cup cooked	120
Orange juice, 4 ounces	110

CALCIUM:
Food	% U.S. RDA
Sardines, drained, 3 ounces	35
Almonds, shelled, 1 cup	35
Tofu, bean curd, 8 ounces	29
Turnip greens, 1 cup cooked	25
Rhubarb, 1 cup cooked	20
Salmon, 3 ounces	20
Broccoli, 1 cup cooked	15
Spinach, 1 cup cooked	15
*Beans, dry (most varieties), 1 cup cooked	8

IRON:
Food	% U.S. RDA
Prune juice, 1 cup	60
Tuna fish, canned, 3 ounces	40
*Liver, beef, 3 ounces	40
*Beans, dry (most varieties), 1 cup cooked	30
Tofu, bean curd, 8 ounces	24
Spinach, 1 cup cooked	20
Beef, ground, 3 ounces	15
Sunflower seeds, ¼ cup	15

POTASSIUM: mg.**
Food	mg.
*Beans, dry (most varieties), 1 cup cooked	790
Chestnuts, fresh, shelled, 1 cup	726
Avocado, half medium	725
Prunes, dried, 10 medium uncooked	705
Beans, green, 1 cup cooked	675
Banana, 1 medium	647
Raisins, ½ cup uncooked	625
Carrots, raw, 1 cup sliced	592
Chicken, cooked, 3 ounces	349
Apricots, dried, 10 medium halves	342
Beef, ground, 3 ounces	315

*If able to tolerate
**U.S. RDA for potassium has not been established. Figures shown are milligrams (mg.).

SOURCE: Based on U.S. Department of Agriculture data.

MAKING MILK EASIER TO DIGEST

There are products on the market that may make it possible for you to drink milk and use milk products IF your problem is simple lactose intolerance. However, if you are allergic to milk or suffer from galactosemia, these treated milk products or enzyme tablets can't help you. If you are diabetic, or have had milk removed from your diet for other medical reasons, you should consult your doctor first.

LactAid is a lactase enzyme preparation which makes milk digestible for some persons who are unable to digest lactose, the complex natural sugar. LactAid may do for you what your own body can't do if you are lactose intolerant; that is, separate the lactose into the more digestible sugars, glucose and galactose.

LactAid is a liquid which, when added to milk, can hydrolyze a predictable level of lactose before the milk is consumed. The longer the blended milk stands in the refrigerator, the higher the level of lactose conversion. After twenty-four hours of blending, the milk has had about 70% of the original lactose converted to the more easily digested galactose and glucose. The conversion level can reach 90% after three or four days in the refrigerator. Higher levels of conversion can also be achieved by adding more LactAid or by heating the milk according to the instructions provided.

LactAid treated milk will taste a little sweeter than untreated milk and will also be more perishable. It should always be handled carefully and refrigerated promptly. The treated milk can be used for cooking and baking. LactAid treated milk may also be cultured but LactAid cannot be used to treat other dairy products, such as cheese, yogurt, or buttermilk. Since it is an enzyme that can be destroyed by too much heat, you should follow instructions for its use carefully.

LactAid is produced by the Sugarlo Company. Anyone wishing more information can write to the company at the address shown in the "Product Information Directory" on page 127. They will be pleased to send you a 4-quart treatment trial size for 50¢ in coin or stamps.

Another means of coping with lactose intolerance may be provided by the recently developed lactase tablets, made to be taken orally before or with the consumption of milk or milk products. The Malabar Milk Digestant Tablets, for example, contain 25 mg. lactase and 2 mg. rennin per tablet. One to three tablets (depending on degree of intolerance) are recommended before or during any meal containing milk products. Although some physicians are not convinced of the efficacy of these tablets, they apparently have been effective for some milk intolerants. They may be particularly useful for those traveling and dining away from home. If you intend to use any milk digestant tablet as a hedge against lactose intolerance symptoms, please check with your physician first.

Finally, there is fresh milk that is fortified with the bacteria, "Lactobacillus Acidophilus"; this product is sold (in the dairy case) under the trademark "Sweet Acidophilus". While there are no wholly conclusive research findings at this point, preliminary indications are that this product may ease some of the common problems induced by lactose intolerance: intestinal cramps and diarrhea, for example. Because heat destroys its special properties, however, this product cannot be used in cooking or added to hot beverages. Like all dietary changes, check this one with your doctor first since it is likely that it can be of help only to those who are mildly lactose intolerant.

TOFU: THE VERSATILE SOY CHEESE

If you've wondered how to satisfy the need for calcium in your diet, you may find the answer in tofu, the "cheese" made from curds of soybean milk.

Unlike soy milk, which has a stronger flavor than we have been accustomed to in cow's milk, tofu is almost tasteless. For this reason, it needs careful preparation and seasoning but it can be substituted for cheese, used to extend meat or fish dishes, and used in salads, sandwich fillings or desserts. Its' nutritional value makes it a boon for anyone on a milk-free diet.

Tofu can be purchased fresh in some vegetable markets (where you'll probably find the creamy looking cakes floating in a tub of water) or in health food stores. It is also available canned or vacuum sealed in plastic containers. The method of packaging will determine how long it will stay fresh in your refrigerator or pantry but, once opened, will normally remain fresh for about a week. To ensure that it retains its mild flavor, it should be stored in a container of water in the refrigerator and the water changed daily.

The molded cakes of fresh tofu usually weigh between 6 and 8 ounces while most canned or vacuum sealed packages come in a one pound size. Japanese style tofu is less compact, often lighter in color (like cottage cheese) than the Chinese style which is pressed into firmer, drier cakes.

When preparing to use tofu, it is best to press it gently first to remove as much moisture from it as you can. Just slice, cube, or crumble it as the recipe directs and weight it down. In 15 or 20 minutes the excess moisture will be absorbed by the towels and it will be ready for use.

Living...Without Milk

While there are only a few tofu recipes in this cookbook, its' uses are almost endless. The traditional Japanese way is to dice it and serve it with a variety of highly seasoned sauces for dipping. In our own kitchen, we like to marinate the cubes briefly in a spicy salad dressing, chill well, and serve in tossed salad. And, of course, you'll find dozens of ideas - starting with Sukiyaki - in any good Oriental cookbook.

Brands vary in texture and flavor so, if you aren't "turned on" by your first venture with tofu, try again - the nutrients make it worthwhile. To emphasize its' value, we've included the following comparison chart:

NUTRIENT	3.5% FAT WHOLE MILK 2 cups	Uncreamed COTTAGE CHEESE 1 pound	Soybean TOFU 1 pound
VITAMIN A:	12	1	-
VITAMIN B1:	8	9	17
VITAMIN B2:	50	75	8
CALCIUM:	30	41	58
IRON:	-	10	48
CALORIES:	(320)	(390)	(327)

──── % U.S. RDA ────

*Rounded to nearest %
-Negligible or less than 1%

"The best treatment of allergy to food is to avoid the offending foods in all their forms." Dr. Frederic Speer, Speer Allergy Clinic, Shawnee Mission, Kansas.

SPECIAL HELP for Milk-free Diets

It sounds simple enough. If you or a family member are sensitive to milk, just eliminate milk from the menu and you eliminate the problem.

Unfortunately, it is not that easy. As we have learned, milk comes in a variety of forms, many of which are found in the packaged convenience foods we take for granted. The only solution is to prepare more meals with basic milk-free ingredients. No need to throw out your favorite recipes, however; many can be prepared with equally good results - using the substitute ingredients listed below. These ingredients will be useful, too, in preparing the milk-free convenience foods that begin the recipe section, as well as many of the other recipes in this book.

BUTTER SUBSTITUTE: Several brands of milk-free margarine are listed in the "Product Information Directory" that begins on page 127. However, remember that using the whipped or diet types of margarine as substitute for baking will not give the same results as the hard types.

CHEESE SUBSTITUTE: Soy bean curd, or tofu, is such a nutritionally valuable addition to the milk-free diet that we have included several recipes, as well as a separate chapter of nutrition and preparation information.

CHOCOLATE SUBSTITUTE: Carob powder, processed from the nutritious carob bean, is available as a flavorful substitute for cocoa in baking or beverages. It can be found in most health food stores. However, be sure to buy the plain "powder" rather than the drink "mix," since the latter contains dried milk. Use in the same proportions as you would cocoa. As a substitute for unsweetened chocolate, use 3 tablespoons carob powder and 1 tablespoon milk-free margarine for each 1-ounce square.

MILK AND CREAM SUBSTITUTES:

COCONUT MILK. Fresh coconut milk or canned coconut juice, usually available in 8-ounce cans. (If allergic, avoid brands containing sodium caseinate.) Use for baking or in beverages.

COCONUT MILK BEVERAGES. These ready-to-drink beverages are a milk-free blend of coconut milk and other natural juices added for flavoring and sweetening. They come in a variety of flavors, including plain coconut and Pina Colada and provide a handy base for nutritious "milk" shakes. When used as a baking ingredient, allowance should be made for their sweetness. Coconut milk beverages are usually available in quart bottles at health food stores or supermarkets (where they are sometimes found in the refrigerator case or with the fresh fruit).

"NON-DAIRY" DRY CREAMERS. Read labels carefully; many contain sodium caseinate and some even contain whey. Reconstitute according to directions on the container.

"NON-DAIRY" LIQUID CREAMERS. (If allergic, avoid brands containing sodium caseinate.) May be used successfully in almost any recipe except custards, puddings, and delicate cakes. Use full strength for coffee and rich cream sauce. Dilute two parts creamer to one part water for regular cream sauce, hot cereals, or making cream pies and dessert sauces. Keep some on hand, already diluted with an equal part water, for general use as you would milk - in tapioca, scrambled eggs, milk shakes, or poured over cold cereals. Diluted this way, "non-dairy" liquid creamer has the same number of calories as whole milk but not the nutritional value.

Special Help for Milk-free Diets

SEED AND NUT "MILKS". A variety of seeds and nuts can be prepared to provide a base for beverages. For example, liquify 2 ounces of sesame seeds, raw cashews, or blanched almonds in the blender with 6 ounces of water.

SOY MILK SUBSTITUTES. Isomil, Mullsoy, Neo-Mullsoy, Pro-Sobee, Soyalac, and Similac concentrated liquids. Some of these products, including Mull-Soy and Neo-Mullsoy, will no longer be available after mid-1981 but your doctor or druggist should be able to advise you which brands are still available. Instant powdered soybean, such as Fearn Soya Powder, can be mixed like dried milk and is available in most health food stores. All have a stronger flavor than milk but can be used for drinking or in cooking and have a nutritional value comparable to milk. Be sure to check with your doctor before using any of these products for children under one year old.

"SQUASH "MILK". You will be pleasantly surprised with baking results using this mild flavored vegetable. See the index for the "recipe".

"We must caution persons with milk allergies that since allergies are so highly individualized and can be areas of extreme sensitivity, we recommend that they evaluate these products with their allergist before making any final decision on using them." Rich Products Corporation.

Living...Without Milk

ACKNOWLEDGEMENTS

I would also like to express appreciation to the many food and drug manufacturers who were so quick to respond with information about the ingredients in their products. It was reassuring to realize that they, too, are concerned about any product components that could cause discomfort to their customers. Most of them made it a point to repeat the caution that veteran allergy and intolerance sufferers know so well: "Read the label every time you buy the product".

While the book does provide information about manufacturers and their products as a service to the reader, such mentions do not constitute endorsement of those products.

I have relied on some of the companies for some of the milk-free recipes in this book. These sources are identified by the following abbreviations printed to the right of each recipe:

>The Banana Bunch **(BB)**
>General Foods Corporation **(GF)**
>Rich Products Corporation **(R)**

Jackie Hostage

---

*Indicates that the recipe appears elsewhere in the book. Please check Recipe Index, page 134.

SUPER SUBSTITUTES

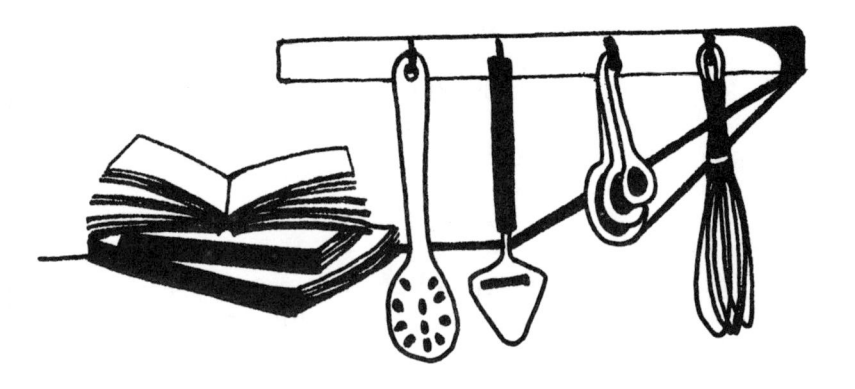

for Convenience Foods

"CHEESE" PASTRY

Here is a delicious way to sneak a few extra nutrients into a variety of pastry recipes. No one will suspect your "secret ingredient".

1 cup milk-free margarine
1 cup tofu, crumbled
2 cups sifted flour
1 tablespoon sugar
¼ teaspoon salt

Drain tofu well to remove excess moisture. Cream the margarine and tofu together until smooth and creamy. Sift together remaining ingredients; work into creamed mixture with pastry cutter or wooden spoon. Mold into a ball; wrap in plastic wrap and chill several hours.

Living...Without Milk

COOKIES: Roll about 1/8" thick; cut into 2½" squares. Place a teaspoonful of tart jam or preserves (cherry or raspberry is particularly good) in the center of each square. Fold corners to center to enclose filling. Bake 15 minutes in a 425° oven or until lightly browned. Cool. Sprinkle with confectioners' sugar. Almost like mini "pop-tarts" and nutritious enough to serve for breakfast.

MINI-MEAT PIES: Brown ½ pound lean ground beef with 1 small chopped onion. Add ½ teaspoon salt, ¼ teaspoon marjoram, dash of pepper and 1 teaspoon dried parsley. (If filling is very moist, add 1 tablespoon bread crumbs or flour.) Cut rolled dough into 4" squares; place about 1 tablespoon filling on each. Fold in half diagonally and press edges with fork tines to seal. Bake as for COOKIES.

WHITE SAUCE

1 tablespoon milk-free margarine
¼ cup flour
¼ teaspoon salt
Dash pepper
½ cup water
1 cup liquid non-dairy creamer

Melt butter in saucepan; blend in flour, salt, pepper, and water. Add creamer. Cook and stir until thickened and sauce comes to a boil.

NOTE: The proportion of margarine to flour is reduced to compensate for the higher fat content of the non-dairy creamer.

To make a thinner sauce, reduce the flour to 2 tablespoons.

CREAM-OF-MUSHROOM SOUP SUBSTITUTE

Here's the answer to all those casseroles you thought you couldn't make without commercial Cream-of-Mushroom soup.

¼ cup minced onion
2 tablespoons minced celery
1 clove garlic, minced
3 tablespoons milk-free margarine
½ pound fresh mushrooms, chopped
¼ cup flour
1 cup chicken or beef broth
    (or 1 cube dissolved in hot water)
1 ½ cups non-dairy creamer
½ teaspoon basil
¾ teaspoon salt

Saute onion, celery, and garlic in margarine until soft. Add mushrooms and brown lightly. Sprinkle flour over, stirring constantly and cooking until all flour is blended in. Gradually add broth, seasonings, and creamer. Bring to boil slowly and simmer two minutes, stirring constantly.

Makes about 2½ cups or the equivalent of two cans of commercial Cream of Mushroom Soup.

NOTE: Recipe doubles easily if you want to make extra for the freezer. Try freezing 1¼ cup single recipe portions in plastic sandwich boxes. When solid, pop out of box, wrap in foil and label. Boxes are ready for re-use. To thaw: Place in saucepan with liquid required for recipe. Heat slowly over low flame or in double boiler.

TOFU "SOUR CREAM"

5 tablespoons non-dairy creamer
1 tablespoon lemon juice
1 cup crumbled tofu

Put ingredients in blender container. Blend until smooth. May be used as a substitute for sour cream in molded salads or well-seasoned dips.

SQUASH "MILK"

Wash and dice yellow squash, leaving skin on but removing seeds. Place slightly more than the amount required for recipe in measuring cup; fill cup with water to just cover squash. Liquify in blender (about 60-90 seconds). Strain. Keeps for several days in the refrigerator; freezes well.

BEER BATTER FOR DEEP FRYING

1 cup self-rising flour
2 egg yolks, beaten
2 egg whites
½ cup flat beer

Combine flour, egg yolks, and beer; stir until batter is smooth. Chill 3-12 hours. Beat egg whites until soft peaks form: fold into batter.

May be used to deep fry chicken, fish, seafood, or vegetables (try whole mushrooms, onion rings, sticks of zucchini or eggplant).

"PACKAGED" BREAD STUFFING

Commercial ready-mix stuffing - free of milk-derived additives - is hard to find but is so handy to have on the pantry shelf. Try this, but be sure that the dried seasonings you use are also additive free.

1 1-pound loaf milk-free bread, ½" cubes
3 tablespoons dried minced onion
3 tablespoons dried parsley
3 tablespoons dried celery leaves
1 tablespoon paprika
2 teaspoons dried sage
1 teaspoon poultry seasoning
2 teaspoons salt
½ teaspoon pepper

Place bread cubes in large plastic or paper bag. Grind seasonings to a powder in blender or pulverize in a mortar. Add seasonings to bread cubes; shake until seasonings cling to bread cubes. TO DRY IN OVEN, place in single layer on cookie sheets and dry about 20 minutes in a 250° oven, stirring occasionally, until crisp and dry but not brown. TO DRY IN MICROWAVE OVEN, place (half recipe at a time) in shallow 8x12-inch glass pan and dry about 8 minutes on "high", stirring every two minutes, until crisp and dry but not brown. Be sure stuffing is completely cool and dry before storing in a tightly closed plastic or glass container.

TO USE: For each 1 cup of stuffing mix, add 1 tablespoon melted milk-free margarine and 2 tablespoons warm water. Toss lightly to combine.

Living...Without Milk

TWO-WAY BREAD STUFFING

Often it is easier to bake the stuffing in a casserole rather than stuffing the poultry. This recipe gives you that option. Will stuff a 4-pound bird or fill a 1½-quart casserole.

⅓ cup milk-free margarine
¼ cup minced onion
4 cups day-old milk-free bread, ½-inch cubes
½ cup chopped celery (with leaves)
1 teaspoon salt
¼ teaspoon pepper
1 teaspoon sage
¼ teaspoon poultry seasoning
½ cup water (optional)

Cook onion in melted margarine until yellow. Add to bread, celery, and seasonings in large bowl; toss lightly. Use to stuff bird. If oven baking is preferred, add liquid and mix gently. Pack lightly in baking pan; cover. Bake along with roast during last 30 to 40 minutes.

"WILD" RICE STUFFING (GF)

1⅓ cups Minute Rice
¼ cup milk-free margarine
¼ pound mushrooms, finely chopped (about 1½ cups)
1¼ cups finely chopped celery and leaves
¼ cup finely chopped onion
1½ teaspoons salt
¼ teaspoon marjoram
Dash of pepper
Pinch of sage
Pinch of thyme
1⅓ cups water
⅓ cup chopped pecans

Saute rice in margarine over medium heat until golden brown, stirring frequently. Add remaining ingredients, except pecans. Bring quickly to a boil over high heat; then simmer 2 minutes, fluffing rice gently with a fork once or twice. Remove from heat and add pecans. Fluff lightly with a fork. Spoon stuffing into poultry. (Do not pack tightly.) Roast at once.

Makes about 4 cups or enough for a 3-to 5-pound chicken - or use in pheasant or Cornish hens.

SEASONED BREAD CRUMBS

Stale milk-free italian bread
1 teaspoon marjoram or oregano
½ teaspoon thyme
½ teaspoon paprika

Grate bread in blender or on hand grater. Add remaining ingredients to 1½ cups of the bread crumbs combining thoroughly by shaking well or whirling in blender. Save any leftover crumbs for PLAIN BREAD CRUMBS.

MINI-CROUTONS

4 cups ¼" cubes fresh milk-free bread
   (about 5 slices white and 3 slices rye)
2 tablespoons oil
1 tablespoon dried parsley
¾ teaspoon garlic salt
1 teaspoon dried minced onion
½ teaspoon each: oregano and paprika
¼ teaspoon each: thyme, basil, pepper

Toast bread cubes in shallow baking pan or on cookie sheet 30 minutes in a 300° oven. Cool slightly. Drizzle with oil; stir in spices, mixing well. Cool before storing in airtight containers. Sprinkle on salads.

FRESH CROUTONS

2 cups ½-inch white milk-free bread cubes
2 tablespoons oil
1 clove garlic (optional)

Use firm type bread if available. Heat oil in heavy skillet; saute bread cubes with garlic over medium heat until golden on all sides. Remove garlic. Drain cubes on paper towels.

Here is a variety of salad dressings for those times when you can't find a commercial product that doesn't contain blended spices or monosodium glutamate...

BOILED SALAD DRESSING

1 egg, slightly beaten
⅓ cup sugar
1 ½ tablespoons flour
½ teaspoon dry mustard
⅔ cup water
⅓ cup vinegar
2 tablespoons milk-free margarine
1 teaspoon salt
¼ teaspoon pepper

Combine all ingredients; boil until thickened. Good for potato salad; for best flavor, combine ingredients while still warm; chill. (Crisp, fried bacon, crumbled makes a complementary addition.) May also be beaten into mayonnaise to vary the flavor or decrease the proportion of oil.

PLAIN SALAD DRESSING

¾ cup salad oil
¼ cup vinegar or lemon juice
½ teaspoon salt
Dash pepper
1 tablespoon sugar
1 clove garlic, mashed

Combine ingredients in jar and shake well.

ITALIAN SALAD DRESSING

1 tablespoon sugar
1 teaspoon salt
½ teaspoon dry mustard
½ teaspoon paprika
½ teaspoon oregano
1 clove garlic, minced
¼ cup onion, finely chopped
¼ cup wine vinegar
¼ cup catsup
¾ cup salad oil

Combine dry ingredients in jar and mix well. Add remaining ingredients; shake well. Chill.

FRESH STRAWBERRY DRESSING

This one is perfect for fruit salads.

¾ cup sliced ripe strawberries
2 tablespoons light corn syrup
½ cup mayonnaise

Mash strawberries together with corn syrup. Add mayonnaise, stirring until well blended. Chill.

BLENDER MAYONNAISE

1 egg
1/8 teaspoon white pepper
1/8 teaspoon paprika
¼ teaspoon dry mustard
1 teaspoon sugar
1 tablespoon lemon juice
1 tablespoon salad vinegar
½ teaspoon salt
1 cup pure corn oil

Have all ingredients at room temperature. Put egg, seasonings, lemon juice, vinegar and ¼ cup of the oil in blender container, cover and turn to blend. Immediately remove center cap and pour in remaining oil in a slow, steady stream. If necessary, stop blender occasionally and use rubber spatula to keep mixture moving into blades. Process until thick and smooth.

NOTE: Homemade mayonnaise does not keep as long as commercial mayonnaise so plan to use within a week and keep refrigerated.

TARTAR SAUCE

½ cup mayonnaise
1 teaspoon dried parsley
2 teaspoons sweet pickle relish
2 teaspoons capers
1 teaspoon minced onion

Combine all ingredients; chill to blend flavors.

STANDARD RECIPES YOU CAN USE

A word about the recipes in this book. Like any specialty cookbook, this one was created to serve a special need: creamy desserts and saucy foods that can satisfy that desire for something rich and "gooey" that seems to be even more urgent when you are on a milk-free diet and know it's a "no-no". Therefore, this is not a complete cookbook and lacks many of the recipes that make up the bulk of plain, nutritious, everyday cooking. Milk-free cooking requires more "cooking from scratch" so here are a few suggestions for recipes found in most cookbooks; usually they are milk-free or easily adjusted.

BAKED BEANS: substitute maple syrup for molasses.

BREADS AND ROLLS: Italian, potato water, fruit/nut tea loaves, breadsticks.

CAKES: Angel food, sponge, applesauce or fruit.

CANDIES: Marshmallows, nougats, fruit jellies, popcorn balls, divinity.

COOKIES: Most require so little milk that fruit juice or "non-dairy" creamer can be substituted.

FROSTINGS: "Seven Minute" or marshmallow, fruit glazes. Use milk-free margarine and juice, coffee, or "non-dairy" creamer in Buttercream type frostings.

FRUIT: Pies, pastries, cobblers, baked apples, stewed fruit, salads, frozen ices.

Living...Without Milk

MEAT LOAVES: Substitute tomato juice, bouillon, or chopped, canned tomatoes for milk. Use milk-free bread, oatmeal, or tapioca.

PIES: Lemon or Orange Meringue, some Chiffon pies, most fruit pies.

SALADS: Fruit, vegetable, "Three Bean", coleslaw with mayonnaise, carrot and raisin, Waldorf. For "chef's salad", substitute quartered hard boiled eggs or milk-free bologna for the cheese. Molded gelatin salads using fruits or vegetables.

SANDWICHES: Chicken, tuna, milk-free cold cuts, barbecued meats.

STUFFINGS: Rice, Kasha, or milk-free cornbread as a change from milk-free bread.

TAPIOCA: made with fruit juice.

ZABAGLIONE: A delicious milk-free dessert. Good served over fresh fruit or berries.

ADUSTING RECIPES: While the fat and sugar content of the "non-dairy" creamers make them unsatisfactory for delicate cakes, you may be able to continue using some of your favorite cake recipes by substituting a combination of water, extra egg, and oil for the milk called for in the recipe. Break one egg in measuring cup; add two tablespoons oil; fill cup with water to make two cups. Blend ingredients well and measure out amount needed to replace milk in recipe.

THE BETTER BREAKFAST

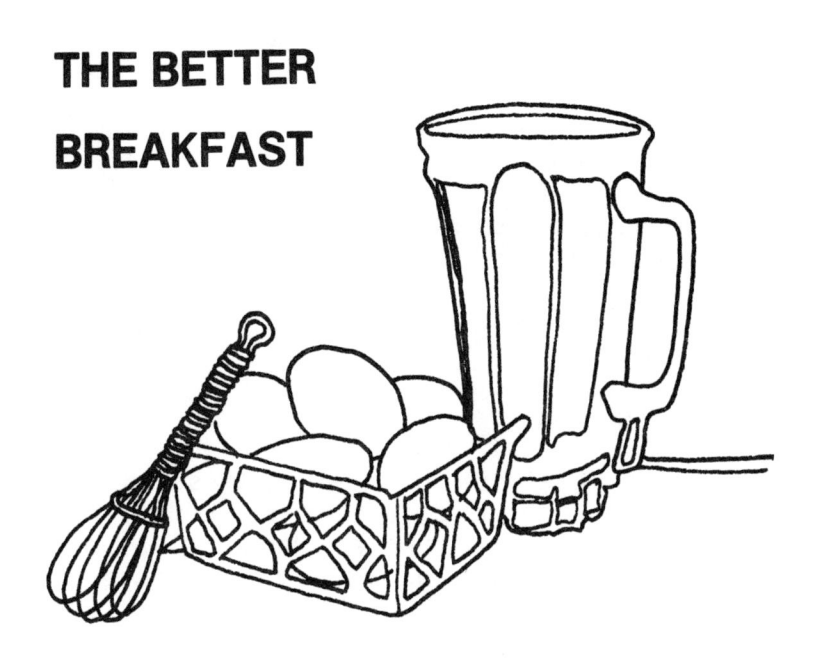

GRAPEFRUIT SURPRISE

Nutritious enough for breakfast; special enough for dessert.

2 grapefruit
1 cup sliced strawberries
2 tablespoons sugar

Halve grapefruit and remove sections. Place in bowl with 1 tablespoon of the sugar; cover and refrigerate. Remove inner membrane from grapefruit shells and reserve shells. Combine strawberries with remaining 1 tablespoon sugar. Chill several hours or overnight. When ready to serve, fill reserved shells with grapefruit and spoon strawberries over.

Makes 4 servings.

Living...Without Milk

CREAMY "SHAKE"

½ cup non-dairy creamer
½ cup ice water
1 teaspoon sugar
¼ cup mashed strawberries
1 tablespoon Vanilla Instant Pudding

Shake in jar or blend in blender. Let stand a minute before serving.

Makes 1 serving.

NOTE: In place of the strawberries, try substituting any one of the following: 2 tablespoons strawberry or raspberry jam, 1 tablespoon instant coffee, or 2 tablespoons chocolate or carob syrup.

Packaged product ingredients are like the weather ... always changing. Read the label **every** time you buy a product.

BANANA HULA (BB)

Here's a "banana break" that will boost your potassium intake for the day.

2 ripe bananas
1 can (12 ounces) unsweetened pineapple juice
2 tablespoons sugar
Flaked coconut

In container of electric blender combine bananas, pineapple juice and sugar. Cover and process until smooth. Serve sprinkled with flaked coconut.

Makes 3 servings.

FRESH FRUIT SMOOTHIE

1 cup pineapple juice
1 cup orange juice
1 peach, cut up (optional)
1 banana, cut up
2 cracked ice cubes
1 tablespoon sugar

Omit peach and mash banana if not using blender. Shake in jar or blend in blender.

Makes 3 servings.

GOLDEN EGGNOG

¼ cup non-dairy creamer
1 egg
½ cup orange juice
2 teaspoons sugar

Mix well with egg beater or blend in blender.

Makes 1 serving.

BERRY TASTY SHAKE

½ cup sliced strawberries
1 teaspoon sugar
½ cup grapefruit juice
1 egg white
1 tablespoon wheat germ
2 crushed ice cubes

Place strawberries in blender jar; sprinkle with sugar. Let stand for a few minutes. Add remaining ingredients. Cover and blend until frothy.

Makes 1 serving.

BREAKFAST COOKIES

Combine these cookies with any of the "meals-in-a-glass" for a nutritious breakfast or snack.

1¼ cups unsifted flour
⅔ cup sugar
½ cup Post® Grape-Nuts® Brand Cereal
1 teaspoon baking powder
½ pound bacon, cooked and crumbled
½ cup milk-free margarine
1 egg
2 tablespoons frozen orange juice concentrate, thawed, undiluted
1 tablespoon grated orange peel

Combine dry ingredients; mix well. Add bacon, margarine, egg, orange juice concentrate, and orange peel. Mix until well blended. Drop by level tablespoons 2 inches apart on ungreased baking sheet.

Bake 10-12 minutes in a 350° oven or until edges of cookies are lightly browned but cookies are still soft.

Makes 2½ dozen.

CRANBERRY NUT MUFFINS

1½ cups unsifted flour
½ cup sugar
1 teaspoon baking powder
½ teaspoon salt
½ teaspoon baking soda
⅓ cup chopped nuts
2 tablespoons orange juice
1 tablespoon salad oil
1 egg, slightly beaten
1 8-oz. can whole berry cranberry sauce

Combine dry ingredients. Add remaining ingredients and stir until dry ingredients are evenly moistened. Fill muffin pans ⅔ full. Bake 15-20 minutes in a 400° oven. Makes 12.

ORANGE CRUMB COFFEE CAKE

½ cup firmly packed brown sugar
½ cup finely chopped nuts
½ teaspoon cinnamon
½ teaspoon nutmeg
2 cups sifted flour
3 teaspoons baking powder
1 teaspoon salt
¼ cup granulated sugar
⅓ cup shortening
1 egg, slightly beaten
¾ cup orange juice
2 tablespoons milk-free margarine

Melt margarine and set aside to cool. Combine brown sugar, nuts, and spices; set aside. Combine flour, baking powder, salt, and granulated sugar in bowl; cut in shortening until mixture resembles coarse meal. Add egg and orange juice, stir until blended. Drop mixture by heaping tablespoonfuls into sugar-nut mixture, shaping into balls and coating well. Place balls in greased 8-inch square pan. Sprinkle with remaining sugar mixture and drizzle with the melted margarine.

Bake 30-35 minutes in a 375° oven. Serve warm.

Living...Without Milk

COLD CEREAL

Similar to the Swiss "muesli", this cereal will need little more than a bit of coconut milk or non-dairy creamer to make it a treat. Here is freshness you will not find in a package.

¼ cup rolled rye
3 tablespoons raisins
2 tablespoons chopped almonds
4 tablespoons shredded or flaked coconut
4 tablespoons water
1 small, unpeeled apple, chopped

Combine all ingredients except apple. Cover and refrigerate overnight. When ready to serve, chop apple and stir in.

Makes 2 servings.

NOTE: Vary the ingredients by substituting oat or wheat flakes, wheat germ, walnuts or pecans. Try diced mixed dried fruit, dates, or prunes instead of raisins; fresh pear instead of apple.

HOMEMADE GRANOLA

This is a delicious substitute for the commercial brands which usually contain non-fat dry milk.

4 cups oatmeal (not instant)
½ cup wheat germ
1 cup sunflower seeds
¾ cup nuts, chopped
¾ cup dates and/or raisins
½ cup corn oil
½ cup honey or brown sugar
2 teaspoons vanilla

Combine oatmeal and wheat germ in large bowl. Mix together oil, honey or brown sugar, and vanilla. Drizzle over cereals and mix well; spread on greased baking sheet. Bake 45 minutes in a 225° oven. Stir in remaining ingredients; bake 15 minutes longer.

NOTE: To vary granola to suit your own tastes, change ingredients or amounts. Other nuts or dried fruits can be used, bran, rolled whole wheat, sesame seeds, coconut, or almost any grain, seed, nut, or dried fruit you have on hand.

PUFFED OMELET (CR)

For each serving:
2 eggs
¼ cup Coffee Rich®
Salt and pepper to taste
2 tablespoons milk-free margarine

FILLING: Sauteed mushrooms, bacon, jelly, or catsup

Separate eggs. Add Coffee Rich® and seasonings to yolks; beat until well mixed. Beat the egg whites until stiff. Fold into the yolks. Melt margarine in 8-inch skillet; add eggs. Cook, loosening and lifting the edges until eggs are set but still moist on top. Spread the eggs with filling, reserving some for garnish. With a rubber spatula roll the omelet away from you and make the final roll by turning the omelet onto serving dish. Garnish with reserved filling.

Living...Without Milk

PANCAKES

1¼ cups sifted flour
2½ teaspoons baking powder
2 tablespoons sugar
¾ teaspoon salt
4 eggs, separated
¾ cup water
3 tablespoons milk-free margarine (melted)

Sift together dry ingredients. Combine egg yolks and water; add to dry ingredients mixing only until dry ingredients are moist. Beat egg whites until stiff; fold beaten egg whites and margarine into batter. Cook on lightly greased griddle.

Makes 16 4-inch pancakes using ¼ cup batter each.

MAPLE "BUTTER"

1⅓ cups maple syrup
1 stick milk-free margarine, cold, cut in pieces
1 egg white

Boil maple syrup down to ⅔ cup. Cool slightly. Place in blender. Add margarine and egg white. Blend until creamy and cooled. Great on toast or pancakes.

"CHOCOLATE" SYRUP

1 cup sugar
½ cup cocoa or carob powder
Dash salt
1 cup water
½ teaspoon vanilla

Combine sugar, cocoa or carob powder, and water in saucepan. Bring to boil and simmer 5 minutes or until ingredients are blended. Add vanilla.

APPETIZERS & DIPS

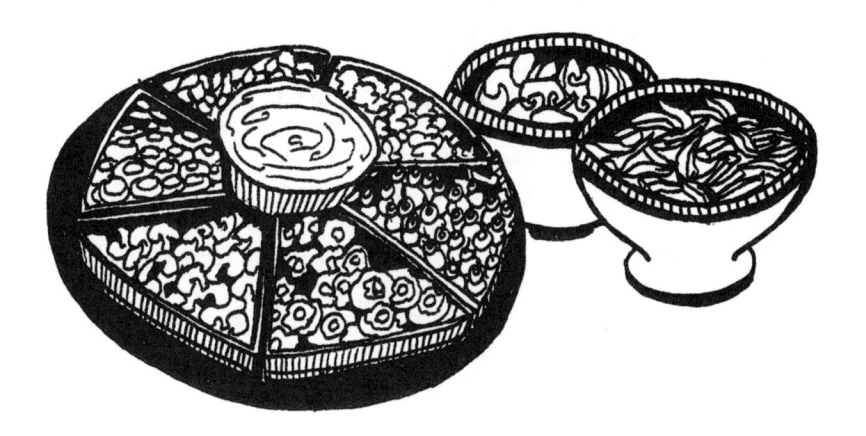

SEAFOOD REMOULADE

2 6-ounce packages frozen cooked shrimp
½ cup celery, finely diced
¼ cup mayonnaise
2 tablespoons sweet pickle relish
2 tablespoons chili sauce
2 teaspoons worcestershire sauce

Thaw and drain shrimp. Combine with remaining ingredients; blend well. Chill.

VARIATION: Substitute 2 6-ounce packages frozen cooked Shrimp and Crab Meat **or** 1 20-ounce can drained chick peas.

NOTE: These make delightful luncheon salads with the addition of more celery and mayonnaise. Serve on lettuce.

BAKED CLAMS OREGANO

4 tablespoons milk-free margarine
2 tablespoons minced onion
1 clove garlic, minced
1 8-ounce can minced clams and juice
1 teaspoon oregano
1 teaspoon parsley flakes
½ cup Seasoned Bread Crumbs*

Saute onion and garlic in margarine until tender. Add remaining ingredients, except bread crumbs; simmer five minutes. Mix in bread crumbs; pile lightly into baking shells. For added "zing", sprinkle lightly with paprika. Fills about 12 2-inch shells.

Bake 15-20 minutes in a 375° oven or until tops are lightly browned.

COCKTAIL MEATBALLS

1 pound ground beef
¼ cup milk-free dry Bread Crumbs*
1 medium onion, minced or grated
1 teaspoon salt
1 egg, beaten
1 cup chili sauce
⅔ cup grape jelly
1 tablespoon lemon juice

Combine ground beef, bread crumbs, onion, salt, and egg; shape into 24-30 small balls. Combine remaining ingredients in shallow saucepan or skillet; heat, stirring until smooth. Drop in meatballs; simmer 20 minutes, covered. If sauce does not completely cover meatballs, turn or baste once during cooking to assure that they brown evenly.

EGGS A LA RUSSE

1 cup mayonnaise
¼ cup catsup
1 tablespoon capers
6 hard-cooked eggs, halved
Lettuce

Combine mayonnaise, catsup, and capers; mix well. Arrange two egg halves on each lettuce-lined plate; top each with dressing to taste.

Makes 6 servings.

COCKTAIL MIX

6 tablespoons milk-free margarine
2 teaspoons worcestershire sauce
1 clove garlic, halved
2 cups Rice Chex®
2 cups Wheat Chex®
2 cups Corn Chex®
1 small bag small pretzels
1 cup salted peanuts

Melt margarine with garlic and let stand a few minutes to absorb flavor. Remove garlic and stir in worcestershire sauce. Pour over remaining ingredients; spread in shallow pan.

Bake 45 minutes in a 250° oven, stirring every 15 minutes.

NOTE: ½ teaspoon garlic powder may replace the garlic clove, if a lactose-free brand is available.

SPICY MARINATED MUSHROOMS

1 pound fresh small mushrooms
½ cup wine vinegar
½ cup salad oil
1 medium onion, thinly sliced
1 clove garlic, minced
1 teaspoon salt
1 tablespoon dried parsley
1 teaspoon prepared mustard
1 tablespoon brown sugar

Rinse mushrooms quickly or wipe with damp paper towel; trim stems. Combine remaining ingredients and bring to boil. Add mushrooms and simmer gently 15 minutes. Chill several hours. Drain just before serving.

MARINATED ARTICHOKES

2 cups artichoke hearts, canned or frozen
2 tablespoons lemon juice
2 tablespoons salad oil
1 tablespoon sugar
1 tablespoon water
1 clove garlic, finely minced
¼ teaspoon dried oregano

If artichoke hearts are frozen, cook according to package directions. Drain. Combine all ingredients in bowl. Cover tightly and chill several hours or overnight. Drain; serve with picks.

NOTE: Leftover marinated mushrooms or artichokes are delicious used in tossed green salad with a plain oil and vinegar dressing.

Appetizers & Dips

ANTIPASTO TRAY

8 thin slices Genoa salami
8 paper-thin slices prosciutto ham
4 hard-cooked eggs, halved
1 cantaloupe, peeled, seeded and cut in thin wedges
Spicy Marinated Mushrooms*, drained
Marinated Artichokes*, drained
Salad or olive oil
Wine vinegar
Salt and pepper

Arrange everything except oil and vinegar on a large serving platter. Accompany with the oil, vinegar, salt and pepper.

TOFU DIP

½ pound tofu
⅓ cup mayonnaise
1 teaspoon prepared mustard
½ teaspoon salt
Dash pepper
½ teaspoon paprika
1 small onion, minced
½ green pepper, finely chopped

Crumble and drain tofu. Mash together with mayonnaise; add seasonings, mix well. Stir in vegetables.

NOTE: Vary the seasonings to suit your taste by adding crushed garlic, tamari sauce, or a dash of turmeric (for a natural yellow color). Other herbs and vegetables, such as celery, carrots, scallions, parsley, dill weed or curry powder, make an interesting change.

Living...Without Milk

TANGY VEGETABLE DIP

1 cup mayonnaise
¼ cup catsup
1 tablespoon chili sauce
2 teaspoons horseradish
1 tablespoon lemon juice
1 clove garlic, minced
Dash tabasco

Combine all ingredients until smooth. Chill for several hours to blend flavors.

NOTE: Reduce or increase the mayonnaise to suit taste.

DIETER'S DELIGHT NIBBLERS

The day before serving, wash **cauliflower** and break into bite-sized flowerets. Clean and cut **carrots, celery,** and **green pepper** into 2-inch sticks. Place vegetables in a large container, alternating with **ice cubes** and sprinkling with 1 tablespoon **salt.** Fill container with cold water, cover tightly, and refrigerate. Just before serving, drain thoroughly and arrange on tray with cleaned, chilled tiny **tomatoes, radishes,** and **scallions.** Serve with TANGY VEGETABLE DIP* .

When inquiring about a product, always ask: "Does this product contain butter, margarine, cheese of any kind, fresh milk, dried or powdered milk, condensed or evaporated milk, buttermilk, fresh or sour cream, yogurt, whey, or any other milk-derived food additive?"

MAIN DISHES

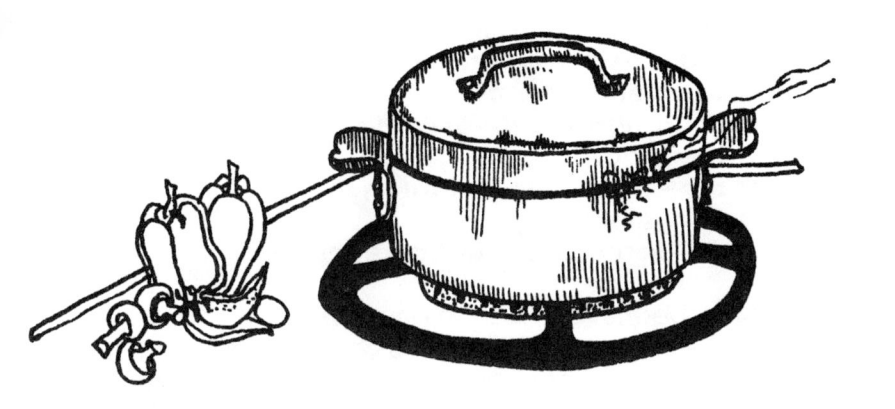

STEAK AND POTATO BROIL

4 beef cube steaks
3 cups diced, cooked potatoes
1 cup diced cucumber
1 tablespoon dried parsley
½ teaspoon salt
Dash pepper
2 tablespoons salad oil
1 tablespoon vinegar
2 medium tomatoes, peeled, halved crosswise

Combine potatoes, cucumber, parsley, salt, pepper, oil, and vinegar; mix well. Spoon into center of foil lined broiler pan. Place tomato halves along edges of pan; sprinkle with additional salt and pepper to taste. Place broiler rack over salad and tomatoes; place in preheated broiler 3-inches from heat and broil 5 minutes. Remove pan from broiler and arrange steaks on center of rack over salad. Broil 5 minutes longer without turning steaks.

Living...Without Milk

BEEF 'N PEPPER STEAK

1 pound beef tenderloin, sliced ¼" thick
2 tablespoons salad oil
1 medium onion, sliced
1 large green pepper, cut in 1" cubes
1 clove garlic, minced
1 cup bouillon or beef broth
1 tablespoon soy sauce
1½ tablespoons cornstarch
¼ cup water
2 small tomatoes, cut into sections

Brown beef in oil. Push to one side. Add onion, pepper, garlic; cook five minutes or until vegetables are softened. Add bouillon, soy sauce, and cornstarch dissolved in the water. Cover; simmer ten minutes or until meat and vegetables are tender. Add tomatoes. Heat through. Serve with rice.

Makes 4 servings.

NOTE: Whole beef tenderloin can be a "bargain" when it's on special because there is so little waste. This is a good recipe to use up the thin end and the trimmings.

SUPER-EASY POT ROAST

3 to 4 pound boneless pot roast
1 envelope onion soup mix

Place meat in center of long sheet of heavy duty foil. Sprinkle all sides of meat with onion soup mix. Close foil, sealing edges with double folds to form airtight package. Place in shallow pan. Bake 3 hours in a 350° oven.

EASY POT ROAST

4 pound boneless pot roast
2 small onions, chopped
1 small carrot, diced
1 stalk celery, diced
2 teaspoons salt
¼ teaspoon pepper
1 bayleaf
½ cup tomato or spaghetti sauce

Brown meat in pan over medium heat; place on large sheet of heavy duty foil. Brown vegetables in same pan; sprinkle on meat along with seasonings. Pour sauce over. Close foil, sealing edges with double folds to form airtight package. Place in shallow pan to catch any leaks.

Bake 3½ hours in a 300° oven **or** 4 hours in a 250° oven.

BARBECUED MEAT LOAVES

1 pound ground beef
1 egg, slightly beaten
2 tablespoons milk-free bread crumbs
1 tablespoon onion, minced
2 tablespoons water
1 teaspoon salt
Dash pepper
⅓ cup catsup
2 tablespoons vinegar
¼ teaspoon worcestershire sauce
½ teaspoon chili powder
1 tablespoon onion, minced

Combine first seven ingredients; form into two loaves. Place in shallow pan. Combine remaining ingredients; spread on loaves.

Bake 35 minutes in 375° oven. Baste once or twice.

Living...Without Milk

BEEF AND VEGETABLE CASSEROLE

1 pound ¼-inch thick roundsteak (or cubed steaks)
1 teaspoon salt
¼ teaspoon pepper
¼ teaspoon paprika
Flour
2 tablespoons shortening
1 medium onion, sliced
3 medium potatoes, sliced
1 cup canned tomatoes

Cut meat into serving pieces. Sprinkle with salt, pepper, and paprika; dredge with flour. Brown in shortening. Place in 1½-quart casserole; add onion and potatoes. Sprinkle with additional salt and pepper to taste. Top with tomatoes.

Bake, covered, 1½ hours in a 350° oven.

Makes 4 servings.

OVEN BEEF RAGOUT

2 pounds beef, cut for stew
3-4 carrots, cut in 1-inch pieces
1 cup chopped celery
2 onions, sliced
3-4 potatoes, pared and cut up
1 16-ounce can tomatoes
1 8-ounce can tomato sauce
1 clove garlic
¼ cup Minute® Tapioca
1 tablespoon sugar
½ cup dry red wine (optional)
1 cup sliced water chestnuts
¼-½ pound sliced fresh mushrooms

Main Dishes

Combine all ingredients except water chestnuts and mushrooms in Dutch oven or large casserole. Cover.

Bake 5 hours in a 250° oven. Add water chestnuts and mushrooms during last hour of baking. Season to taste.

QUICK SAVORY MEAT LOAF (GF)

2 pounds ground beef
1/3 cup Minute® Tapioca
1/3 cup finely chopped onion
1 1/2 teaspoons salt
1/4 teaspoon pepper
1/4 teaspoon savory (optional)
1 12-ounce can tomatoes, mashed

Combine all ingredients, mixing well. Spoon into 9x5-inch loaf pan. Press lightly.

Bake 1 to 1 1/4 hours in a 350° oven.

PORK CHOP SKILLET DINNER

4 pork chops
3 medium onions, sliced
3 raw potatoes, sliced
dry mustard
1 1/2 cups drained canned tomatoes

Brown chops in pan and remove. Rub thoroughly with dry mustard. Brown the onions in the same pan; cover with the sliced potatoes, the pork chops. Cover with the tomatoes; season to taste with salt and pepper. Simmer for one hour or until chops and potatoes are tender.

Makes 4 servings.

OVEN BARBECUED CHICKEN

4 pounds cut-up chicken broiler parts
1 large onion, sliced
⅔ cup catsup
⅓ cup vinegar
4 tablespoons milk-free margarine
1 clove garlic, minced
1 teaspoon salt
1 teaspoon rosemary
¼ teaspoon dry mustard

Place chicken skin side down in single layer on shallow, greased pan. Top with onion slices. Combine remaining ingredients; heat to boiling. Pour over chicken.

Bake for 30 minutes in a 400° oven; turn; baste; bake 30 minutes longer or until chicken is brown and tender.

SKILLET HERB CHICKEN

3 pounds chicken parts, cut-up
¼ cup flour
¾ teaspoon salt
¼ teaspoon pepper
¼ cup shortening
1¼ cups Cream of Mushroom Soup Substitute*
½ cup water (part white wine, if desired)
1 medium onion, sliced
½ teaspoon thyme

Coat chicken with flour and seasonings; brown in heated shortening in skillet. Add soup, water; top with onion slices, thyme. Simmer, covered, basting often for 30 minutes or until tender.

Makes 4 servings.

Main Dishes

VERSATILE BAKED CHICKEN

4 small chicken breasts, split and boned
½ cup milk-free margarine
2 tablespoons flour
1 cup cornflake crumbs
1 teaspoon salt
1 teaspoon rosemary or oregano, crumbled

Melt margarine and blend in flour until smooth. Dip chicken pieces in margarine mixture and coat well with combined crumbs and seasonings. Place on shallow baking pan and refrigerate if not baking immediately.

Bake 45-60 minutes in 350° oven.

NOTE: Crumbs will adhere better and be crisper if skin is removed from chicken. Any type of chicken parts can be used; if using boneless cutlets, use the shorter baking time but use the longer baking time when using large cutlets or bone-in chicken parts.

Mayonnaise or barbecue sauce may be substituted for the margarine and flour or a large clove of garlic, crushed, can be added to the margarine mixture. Seasoned dry bread crumbs or crushed potato chips can replace the cornflake crumbs.

A very adaptable recipe that is equally delicious hot or cold and is particularly festive served with a sauce made by heating 1¼ cups CREAM-OF-MUSHROOM SOUP SUBSTITUTE* 'with ½ cup dry white wine.

Living...Without Milk

CHICK-A-BOBS

1 pound boneless chicken breasts, skinned
1 8-ounce can pineapple chunks
1 clove garlic, crushed
2 tablespoons soy sauce
1 tablespoon dry sherry
1 tablespoon salad oil
8 whole mushrooms
8 small canned or partially cooked onions
8 cherry tomatoes
1 green pepper, cut in 1-inch squares

Cut chicken into 1½-inch cubes. Drain pineapple, reserving liquid. Combine garlic, soy sauce, sherry, oil, and 2 tablespoons of the reserved pineapple juice. Pour over chicken. Marinate several hours or overnight in refrigerator. Drain chicken, reserving marinade. Divide remaining ingredients equally and thread onto 4 skewers. Brush with marinade. Broil 6 inches from heat for 10 minutes; turn, baste and broil 8 minutes longer, basting with additional marinade occasionally. Sprinkle with salt and pepper.

CHICKEN-MACARONI CASSEROLE

3 pounds chicken parts, cut-up
¼ cup flour
½ teaspoon salt
¼ teaspoon pepper
¼ cup cooking oil
½ cup chopped onion
¼ cup chopped green pepper
1 clove garlic, minced
3 carrots, sliced
3 stalks celery, sliced
1 16-ounce can tomato sauce
1 cup water
1½ cups elbow macaroni, uncooked

Shake chicken in plastic bag containing flour, salt, and pepper. Brown in heated oil in skillet. Remove from pan and lightly saute onion, pepper, and garlic. Add remaining ingredients, except macaroni, and simmer 10 minutes. Put macaroni in large, lightly greased casserole; cover with chicken pieces, pour sauce over all. Cover.

Bake 1½ hours in a 325° oven.

SWEET AND SOUR CHICKEN

1 pound boneless chicken breast
2 tablespoons bacon fat
1 20-ounce can pineapple tid-bits
⅓ cup apple cider vinegar
¼ cup brown sugar
½ cup water
2 tablespoons cornstarch
½ teaspoon salt
1 tablespoon soy or tamari sauce
¾ cup thinly sliced green pepper
½ cup thinly sliced onion

Cut chicken breast into 1-inch pieces. Heat bacon fat in large skillet and brown chicken until golden brown on all sides. Drain pineapple, reserving syrup. Combine reserved syrup, vinegar, brown sugar, water, cornstarch, salt and soy or tamari sauce. Bring to boil in medium size pan; cook until clear and slightly thickened. Add chicken; cook, covered, over low heat 45 minutes or until chicken is tender. Refrigerate. When ready to serve, heat chicken mixture over low heat until steaming hot. Add green pepper, onion, and pineapple tid-bits; cook 5 minutes.

Makes 4 servings. Rice and Chinese noodles go well with this.

Living...Without Milk

CHICKEN NORMANDY

2 whole chicken breasts, split
1 tablespoon salad oil
½ cup dry white wine
1 clove garlic, minced
1 small onion, grated
½ teaspoon salt
½ teaspoon pepper
½ teaspoon celery salt
¼ teaspoon each dried thyme, rosemary, marjoram

Rinse chicken breasts and place in plastic bag. Combine remaining ingredients and pour over chicken; marinate in refrigerator for several hours, turnng occasionally. Place chicken skin side down in shallow pan; pour marinade over.

Bake 60 minutes in a 375° oven, turning once and basting several times.

POT ROASTED CHICKEN

4 cups stale milk-free bread cubes
2 small onions, minced
1 small apple, diced
1 teaspoon salt
½ teaspoon poultry seasoning
4 tablespoons milk-free margarine
2 tablespoons water
2 2½-3-pound chickens, whole
¼ cup shortening
1 clove garlic, minced
1 teaspoon summer savory or rosemary
⅔ cup dry white wine or vermouth

Main Dishes

Combine bread, onion, apple, salt, and poultry seasoning. Melt margarine in the water; pour over stuffing ingredients; toss lightly. Use to stuff chickens. In large Dutch oven, or electric fry pan with domed lid brown chickens on all sides in shortening. Add remaining ingredients. Cover tightly. Simmer 1-1½ hours.

BAKED STUFFED CHICKEN BREASTS

4 small whole boneless chicken breasts, skin left on
2 cups "Packaged" Bread Stuffing*
2 tablespoons milk-free margarine, melted
½ teaspoon salt
¼ teaspoon paprika
1 cup chicken broth or bouillon
2 tablespoons milk-free margarine
1½ tablespoons flour
¼ teaspoon dried parsley
¼ cup sherry

Prepare bread stuffing as directed in recipe. Stuff chicken breasts, wrapping the skin around the stuffing. Place on shallow baking pan; drizzle with melted margarine; sprinkle with salt and paprika.

Bake 1 hour in a 375° oven. (Bake sweet potatoes alongside for the last 45 minutes, if desired.)

Meanwhile, prepare sauce. Melt margarine in small pan; stir in flour. Add broth and dried parsley. Simmer 3 minutes or until smooth and thickened. Add sherry; reheat. Serve with baked chicken breasts.

NOTE: One container of CREAM-OF-MUSHROOM SOUP SUBSTITUTE* heated with ½ cup dry white wine makes a delicious sauce, if preferred.

OVEN FRIED FISH FILLETS

1 ½ pounds cod or haddock, fresh or frozen
2 tablespoons lemon juice
¼ cup flour
½ teaspoon salt
½ cup milk-free margarine, melted
1 cup cornflake crumbs

Thaw fillets if frozen. Rinse, pat dry, and cut into serving portions. Combine lemon juice, flour, salt, and margarine, stirring into a smooth paste. Dip fish in paste; coat well with cornflake crumbs. Arrange in single layer on foil-lined baking pan.

Bake 20 minutes in a 400° oven or until fish flakes easily with a fork.

Makes 6 servings.

SEVEN SEAS CASSEROLE

1 ¼ cups Cream of Mushroom Soup Substitute*
1 ¼ cups water (part creamer, if desired)
¼ teaspoon salt
¼ cup chopped onion (optional)
1 ⅓ cups Minute® Rice
1 6 ½ ounce can tuna, salmon, or lobster
1 box thawed frozen peas

Combine soup, water, onion, and salt; bring to boil. Pour half into greased 1 ½ quart casserole. In layers, add Minute® Rice, seafood, peas. Pour over remaining soup; sprinkle with paprika, if desired. Cover.

Bake 20 minutes in a 375° oven.

CREAMY SCALLOP CASSEROLE

1 pound bay scallops
      (or cut up sea scallops)
1 egg yolk, beaten
¼ cup liquid non-dairy creamer
1 teaspoon lemon juice
2 tablespoons vermouth (or white wine)
1 tablespoon onion, minced
½ teaspoon salt
Dash pepper
¾ cup fresh milk-free bread crumbs
1 tablespoon milk-free margarine, melted

Place scallops in bottom of shallow 1-quart baking dish. Combine egg yolk, creamer, lemon juice, vermouth and seasonings; pour over scallops. Combine bread crumbs and margarine and sprinkle over top of casserole.

Bake 30 minutes in a 350° oven; raise heat to 450° for a few minutes more to brown crumbs.

CRUNCHY TUNA BAKE

1 6½-ounce can tuna, drained
4 ounces wide egg noodles
1¼ cups Cream of Mushroom Soup Substitute*
1 4-ounce package potato chips
2 hard cooked eggs (optional), quartered

Cook noodles as directed on package and drain well. Reserve enough potato chips for top of casserole; crush remaining chips and cover bottom of shallow 1½ quart casserole. Combine remaining ingredients; turn into casserole; top with chips.

Bake 20 minutes in 350° oven or until bubbly.

BAKED FISH CREOLE

1 pound fish fillets
1 small onion, finely chopped
½ green pepper, finely chopped
1 large tomato, peeled and chopped
½ teaspoon salt
Dash pepper
¼ teaspoon each dried rosemary, marjoram, thyme
1 tablespoon salad oil

Cut fillets in serving pieces; place in greased shallow baking dish. Combine remaining ingredients and spread over fish.

Bake 20 minutes, uncovered, in a 400° oven.

TOFU MANICOTTI

8 uncooked manicotti shells
1 small onion, minced
1 clove garlic, minced
1 tablespoon milk-free margarine
2 cups crumbled tofu (about two cakes)
2 teaspoons dried parsley
1 egg, slightly beaten
1 quart tomato sauce with meat
          (preferably homemade)

Cook manicotti shells according to package directions until tender; drain; allow to cool. Crumble and measure tofu; place on paper towel and let excess moisture drain while preparing remaining ingredients. Meanwhile, saute onion and garlic in margarine until onion is transparent. Combine sauteed onions and garlic, tofu, parsley, egg, and salt and pepper to taste. Fill shells with mixture. Pour half of the tomato sauce in the bottom of a shallow baking dish. Place stuffed shells in dish in a single layer; pour remaining

Main Dishes

sauce over the manicotti. Cover with aluminum foil. (May be refrigerated at this point for baking later if desired.)

Bake, covered, 40-45 minutes in a 350° oven.

NOTE: For family members not on a lactose-free diet, sliced mozzarella cheese may be used on their portions. After baking, top part of the manicotti with the cheese, continue baking, uncovered, until cheese melts and is bubbly, about 5 minutes.

TUNA-TOFU LOAF

1 6½-ounce can tuna, drained
3 eggs, slightly beaten
¼ cup milk-free dry bread crumbs
1 small onion, minced
1 tablespoon dried parsley
½ cup tomato sauce
½ teaspoon salt
½ teaspoon baking powder
1 cup tofu, crumbled (about ¼ pound)

Press tofu to remove excess moisture. Crumble or shred and measure; place on paper towel to drain any additional moisture while preparing remaining ingredients. In mixing bowl, flake tuna and combine with remaining ingredients except tofu. Fold in tofu gently but thoroughly. Pour into greased 8x4-inch loaf pan, cover, and refrigerate for at least 1 hour (but no longer than 1 day).

Bake uncovered, for 50 to 60 minutes in a 350° oven or until brown.

NOTE: For plain tuna loaf, substitute an additional can of tuna for the tofu.

CELERY-DILL SAUCE* or CREAM-OF-MUSH-ROOM SOUP SUBSTITUTE* (thinned with a little white wine) complement this very well.

SPINACH TOFU QUICHE

A real bonanza of all the nutrients that are hard to find in a milk-free diet.

1 9-inch unbaked pie shell
½ pound tofu
1 10-ounce package frozen, chopped spinach
1 medium onion, chopped
1 tablespoon dried parsley
1 teaspoon dried dill weed
8 slices bacon (about ½ pound)
3 eggs
¾ cup non-dairy creamer
¼ cup water
1 tablespoon flour
1 teaspoon salt
¼ teaspoon pepper
Dash Tabasco

Rinse and crumble tofu; place on paper towel and let excess moisture drain while preparing other ingredients. Cook spinach, according to package directions; drain well, pressing out excess moisture. Fry bacon until crisp; crumble into small pieces; drain on paper towel. Saute onion in remaining bacon fat until golden; remove from pan with slotted spoon to drain excess bacon fat. Combine spinach, onion, parsley, and dill week; gently mix in tofu. Sprinkle bacon in bottom of pie shell; top with tofu mixture. Combine remaining ingredients; beat just enough to mix thoroughly; pour over ingredients in pie shell.

Bake 15 minutes on lower rack of 450° oven; reduce temperature to 300°. Bake 30 minutes longer or until custard is set.

NOTE: Refrigerated or frozen leftovers reheat very well; in fact, the flavor is improved.

Main Dishes

HERBED MUSHROOM OMELET

½ pound mushrooms, rinsed and dried
2 tablespoons onion, minced
4 tablespoons milk-free margarine
¼ teaspoon thyme or tarragon, crumbled
8 eggs
½ teaspoon salt
Dash black pepper

Slice mushrooms. Heat margarine in large skillet. Add mushrooms and herb; saute five minutes, stirring occasionally. Beat eggs with salt and pepper and pour over mushrooms in skillet. Cook over medium heat. Loosen set portion with spatula and tilt pan to let uncooked portion run underneath. Cook until set but not dry.

SPANISH OMELET

½ cup chopped onion
½ cup chopped green pepper
½ cup thinly sliced celery
1 large tomato, diced and drained
¼ teaspoon sugar
salt and pepper
6 eggs, beaten
3 tablespoons milk-free margarine

Saute onion and pepper in 2 tablespoons of the margarine, about 8 minutes or until almost tender but not brown. Add celery and tomato; sprinkle with seasonings. Cover and cook slowly about 5 minutes or until celery is tender. Uncover, raise heat and cook to evaporate juices. Add remaining margarine; pour in eggs and cook, stirring until eggs have set.

Living...Without Milk

CHILI CON CARNE

1 pound ground beef
1 large onion, sliced
2 tablespoons salad oil
1 clove garlic, crushed
1 green pepper, chopped
1 28-ounce can tomatoes, broken up
1½ teaspoons salt
1 bay leaf, crushed
1 tablespoon chili powder
1 20-ounce can dark red kidney beans, drained
½ cup water or red wine

Brown the onion and garlic in the salad oil. Add beef and green pepper; brown, stirring as the meat cooks. Add the tomatoes, salt, bay leaf, and chili powder. Cover and simmer 2 hours. Add the kidney beans and water or wine. Heat.

NOTE: Serve over rice for a "complete protein". While this seems starchy, the rice is a nice foil for the chili.

SUMMERTIME SPAGHETTI

4 cups peeled, diced fresh tomatoes
¼ cup salad or olive oil
3 cloves garlic, halved
¼ cup fresh, chopped parsley
1 tablespoon dried basil
1 teaspoon dried oregano
2 teaspoons salt
¼ teaspoon pepper
1 pound spaghetti

Combine all ingredients except spaghetti; let stand at room temperature for 1 or 2 hours. Remove garlic. When ready to serve, cook and drain spaghetti. Pour mixture over; toss well.

ACCOMPANIMENTS

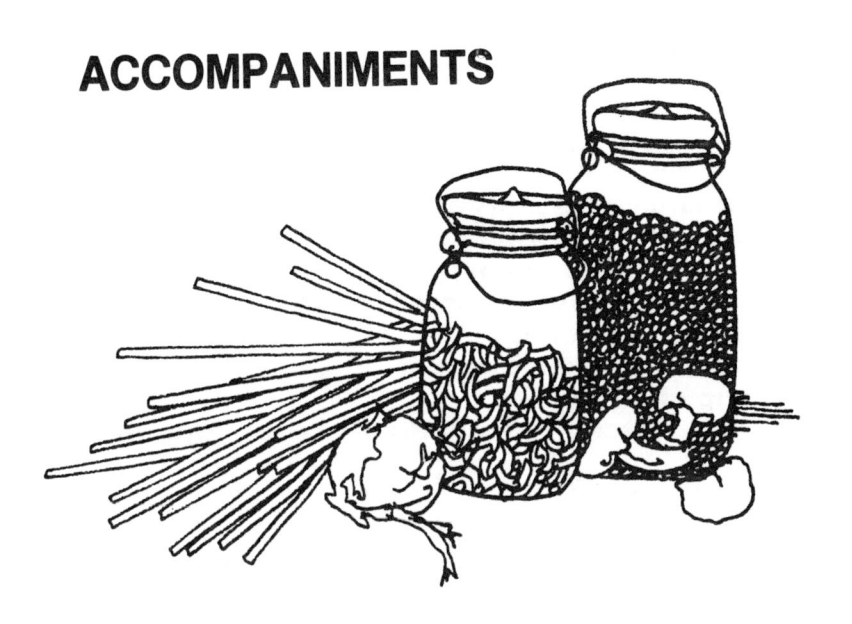

CRUNCHY POTATO CASSEROLE

Similar to potato "kugel", this makes a nice change and can bake right along with the roast.

6 medium potatoes, peeled
4 eggs
½ cup milk-free margarine, melted
1 medium onion, grated
1 teaspoon salt (or to taste)
1/8 teaspoon pepper

Grate potatoes coarsely into a bowl containing 1 or 2 cups of hot water to keep them from turning dark. Beat the eggs lightly; stir in the margarine, onions, and seasonings. Drain potatoes well, pressing to remove excess moisture. Combine with the egg mixture. Pour into a shallow 2-quart casserole.

Bake 1½ hours in a 350° oven or until potatoes are very crisp and brown.

SCALLOPED POTATOES

2 pounds potatoes, peeled and thinly sliced
¼ cup flour
¼ cup milk-free margarine
⅓ cup finely chopped onion
¼ cup diced green pepper
1 cup sliced mushrooms (optional)
Salt and pepper to taste
1 ½ cups chicken broth
¼ cup sherry
½ cup lactose-free cheddar cheese (optional)

Pat potatoes dry; toss with flour. In 2-quart, shallow, greased casserole, alternate layers of potatoes, onion, pepper, mushrooms, and seasonings; dot each layer with some of the margarine. Pour broth and wine over. Cover. Bake 45 minutes in a 375° oven. Uncover; sprinkle with cheese, if desired. Bake an additional 30 minutes, uncovered.

SWEET POTATO BAKE

4 medium sweet potatoes (2 pounds)
2 tablespoons milk-free margarine, soft
2 egg yolks, slightly beaten
¼ cup sugar
½ teaspoon salt
¼ cup orange juice
1 teaspoon grated orange rind
2 egg whites, stiffly beaten

Cook potatoes in boiling water to cover until tender. Remove skins and mash potatoes well. Add remaining ingredients, except egg whites; blend well. Fold stiffly beaten egg whites into potato mixture. Spoon into greased 1-quart casserole or souffle dish.

Bake 35 minutes in a 400° oven until puffed and lightly browned.

Accompaniments

SAVORY LEMON RICE (GF)

½ clove garlic, minced
2 tablespoons milk-free margarine
1⅓ cups Minute® Rice
1⅓ cups chicken broth
½ teaspoon salt
2 tablespoons chopped parsley
1 tablespoon lemon juice
1 teaspoon grated lemon rind

Saute garlic in margarine until golden brown. Stir in rice, broth, and salt. Bring quickly to boil over high heat. Cover, remove from heat, and let stand 5 minutes. Add parsley, lemon juice, and rind and fluff with a fork before serving. Serve with fish, seafood, or chicken.

Makes 4 servings.

BARBECUE RICE (GF)

1⅓ cups water
½ teaspoon salt
¼ teaspoon tabasco sauce
1 teaspoon prepared mustard
2 tablespoons minced onion
2 tablespoons chili sauce
2 tablespoons milk-free margarine
1⅓ cups Minute® Rice

Combine all ingredients except rice in saucepan. Bring to a boil. Stir in rice. Cover, remove from heat, and let stand 5 minutes. Fluff with fork before serving.

Makes 4 servings.

Living...Without Milk

SAVORY OVEN-BAKED RICE

1 small onion, finely chopped
⅓ cup chopped celery
¼ pound mushrooms, chopped
3 tablespoons oil
1½ cups uncooked regular rice
3 envelopes instant chicken broth
¼ teaspoon sage
¼ teaspoon basil
3½ cups boiling water

Saute vegetables in oil until almost tender. Combine in 2-quart casserole with rice and seasonings. Pour boiling water over rice; stir with a fork; cover.

Bake 45 minutes in a 350° oven. Fluff up rice with a fork before serving.

NOODLE RING

¼ cup milk-free margarine, melted
1 pound wide noodles
4 eggs, separated
1 teaspoon cinnamon
¼ teaspoon nutmeg
1¼ cups sugar
¼ teaspoon salt
1 cup raisins
½ cup chopped nuts

Cook and drain noodles. Add margarine. Beat egg yolks with sugar; blend in seasonings. Fold lightly into noodles. Beat whites until stiff but not dry; fold into noodle mixture. Pour ⅓ of mixture into greased 2-quart baking dish; sprinkle with half of the raisins and nuts; repeat; add remaining ⅓ of mixture.

Bake 45 minutes in a 325° oven. Unmold or serve from dish.

NOTE: For an easy, no-pot-watching way to cook noodles (or spaghetti), just bring the required amount of water and salt to a full boil. Slowly drop in the noodles so that boiling doesn't stop. Stir and cover tightly. Remove from heat. Let stand 20 minutes.

VEGETARIAN BAKED BEANS

1 pound navy or pea beans
2 medium onions, quartered
½ cup maple syrup or brown sugar
2 tablespoons sweet pickle juice
1 tablespoon salt
2 teaspoons dry mustard
¼ teaspoon pepper

Wash and pick over beans, removing any broken beans or bits of stone. Cover with 3 cups water; soak 8 hours or overnight. Do not drain. Add an additional 2 cups water and the remaining ingredients. Boil, covered about 1 hour or until beans are almost tender.

Pour into bean pot; sprinkle with additional pepper. Bake 6 to 8 hours in a 250° oven, adding additional water, if necessary, after 4 hours. (Use just enough to barely cover beans.) Uncover beans during last half hour of baking.

Makes 6-8 servings.

NOTE: If sweet pickle juice is not available, substitute 2 tablespoons vinegar with a dash each of cloves and cinnamon.

BAKED BEAN CASSEROLE

6 slices bacon, diced
1 large green pepper, diced
2 medium onions, chopped
½ pound mushrooms, chopped
3 1-pound cans pork and beans in tomato sauce
¾ cup chili sauce
⅓ cup prepared mustard
1 cup maple syrup
1½ teaspoons oregano
5 whole cloves
3 bay leaves

Cook bacon until crisp and remove from pan. In remaining fat, saute green pepper, onions, and mushrooms until just tender. Add remaining ingredients; heat on top of stove just long enough to blend flavors. Serve immediately or store in refrigerator and reheat later by baking for 30 minutes in a 400° oven.

SAVORY TOMATOES

4 large, firm tomatoes
2 cups fresh, milk-free bread crumbs
2 tablespoons dried parsley
2 tablespoons chopped onion
½ teaspoon sage or oregano
Dash pepper
¼ cup milk-free margarine, melted

Core tomatoes and halve crosswise. Place cut side up on shallow, greased pan. Combine remaining ingredients; spread on tops of tomatoes.

Bake 10 minutes in a 450° oven.

Makes 8 servings.

Accompaniments

BAKED CARROTS

1 pound carrots, pared
½ teaspoon salt
1 teaspoon sugar
2 tablespoons milk-free margarine

Cut carrots in halves or thirds, depending on size. Place in 1-quart casserole; sprinkle with salt and sugar; dot with margarine.

Bake 1¼ hours in a 325° oven or 1 hour in a 350° oven.

Makes 4 servings.

SAN ANTONIO SPINACH PUDDING (R)

3 eggs
1 cup Coffee Rich®
1 tablespoon grated onion
½ teaspoon salt
¼ teaspoon pepper
1 10-ounce package frozen chopped spinach

Beat eggs until light and lemon colored. Blend in Coffee Rich and seasonings. Cook spinach until just tender, drain, and blend into Coffee Rich-egg mixture. Pour into greased 1-quart casserole.

Bake 45 minutes in a 350° oven or until set and silver knife comes out clean.

Makes 4 servings.

ZUCCHINI PROVENCAL

2 tablespoons milk-free margarine
½ cup onion, chopped
1 clove garlic, minced
4 medium zucchini, unpared
2 tomatoes, peeled and chopped
1 teaspoon salt
Dash pepper
¼ teaspoon oregano

Melt margarine in large skillet. Add onion and garlic; cook five minutes or until tender. Slice zucchini and add to skillet with remaining ingredients. Mix well, sprinkle with seasonings. Cover. Cook over low heat about 15 minutes or just until zucchini is tender but still crisp.

Makes 4 to 6 servings.

GREEN BEANS LUCETTE

1 9-ounce package frozen green beans
1 3½-ounce can french-fried onions
1¼ cups Cream of Mushroom Soup Substitute*
½ cup liquid from beans

Cook green beans according to directions on the package; drain, reserving the ½ cup liquid. Alternate layers of drained beans and onions in shallow 1½ quart baking dish. Mix soup and liquid and pour over vegetables.

Bake 30 minutes in a 350° oven until bubbly.

Makes 4-6 servings.

SOUPS & SALADS

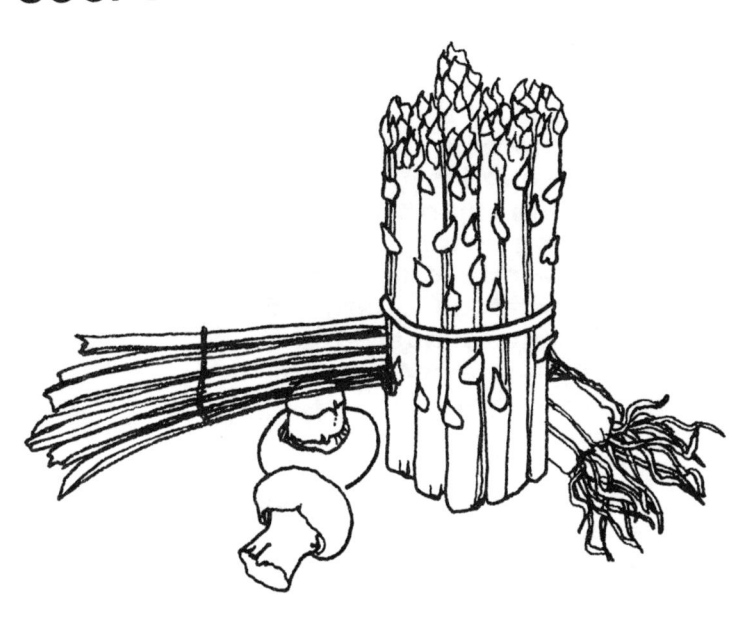

SPEEDY HAMBURGER-VEGETABLE SOUP

½ pound ground beef
1 large onion, chopped
1 clove garlic, minced
4 cups boiling water
4 beef bouillon cubes
1 16-ounce can tomatoes
½ cup diced celery
½ cup diced carrots
½ cup cut green beans
1 tablespoon dried parsley
1 bayleaf
Salt and pepper to taste

Brown ground beef, onion, and garlic lightly, adding oil if necessary. Add remaining ingredients; bring to boil and simmer 30-45 minutes or just until vegetables are done.

Living...Without Milk

BEAN POT SOUP

2 pounds beef for stew, cut in ½-inch pieces
¼ cup flour
2½ teaspoons salt
½ teaspoon pepper
½ teaspoon paprika
3 tablespoons salad oil
4 cups boiling water
6 medium carrots, quartered
4 medium potatoes, quartered
3 medium onions, quartered
1 clove garlic, minced
½ cup sliced celery
2 bay leaves
1 teaspoon sugar
1/8 teaspoon powdered cloves
1 tablespoon lemon juice
1 teaspoon worcestershire sauce

Shake meat in plastic bag with flour, salt, paprika, and pepper to coat well. Brown in oil. Combine with remaining ingredients and place in beanpot. Cover.

Bake 2½ hours in a 350° oven or until meat and vegetables are tender.

MINESTRONE

1 quart leftover beef soup or stew
1 1-pound can tomatoes, chopped
1 cup water or beef bouillon
1 cup shredded cabbage
½ cup elbow macaroni or broken spaghetti
½ teaspoon Italian Seasoning or oregano
1 1-pound can navy, or kidney beans, drained

Remove any potatoes from leftover soup or stew. Add remaining ingredients, except beans, and simmer 15-20 minutes or until macaroni is tender. Add beans; reheat. Adjust seasonings.

Soups & Salads

CREAM OF TOMATO SOUP

1 1-pound can tomatoes
1 tablespoon onion, minced
1 small bayleaf
1 teaspoon sugar
½ teaspoon salt
Dash pepper
¾ cup White Sauce*

In saucepan, combine all ingredients **except** the White Sauce; simmer 10 minutes. (If desired, put through sieve or process in blender.) When ready to serve, stir in White Sauce gradually; heat through. Adjust seasonings and amount of White Sauce to taste.

NOTE: CREAM OF TOMATO SOUP combines very well with leftover CREAM-OF-MUSHROOM SOUP SUBSTITUTE* for a delicious TOMATO-MUSHROOM BISQUE. Thin with additional liquid non-dairy creamer if desired.

CREAM OF CELERY SOUP

1 cup celery, diced
¼ cup onion, finely chopped
1 cup chicken broth or water
1 cup White Sauce*

Cook celery and onion, covered, in chicken broth or salted water until tender (about 15 minutes). Stir in White Sauce. Heat through and season to taste.

Makes 3 servings.

NOTE: To make CELERY-DILL SAUCE, add an additional ½ cup WHITE SAUCE and 1 teaspoon (or to taste) dill weed. Heat through.

GARDEN FRESH VEGETABLE SOUP

3 cups vegetable bouillon made from cubes or packets
1 16-ounce can tomatoes
2 stalks celery with tops, sliced
2 carrots, diced
1 medium onion, chopped
1 medium potato, diced
½ cup fresh or frozen cut green beans
1 teaspoon salt
¼ teaspoon thyme

Drain tomatoes, reserving liquid, and chop. Bring bouillon and tomato liquid to a boil. Add chopped tomatoes and remaining ingredients; simmer 20-30 minutes or just until vegetables are tender. For a heartier flavor, substitute beef bouillon.

VEGETABLE BEAN SOUP

1 pound dry navy beans
2 tablespoons salad oil
4 cups sliced onions
2 cups diced celery
1 cup diced carrots
1 tablespoon minced garlic
2 1-pound cans tomatoes
1 tablespoon salt
4 cups diced zucchini squash
1 tablespoon dried basil
1 tablespoon dried parsley
1 teaspoon oregano

Wash beans; cover with cold water and soak overnight. (Or, simmer 2 minutes; remove from heat; cover and let stand 1 hour.) Don't drain. In large pot, heat oil over medium heat. Add onions, celery, carrots, and garlic; cook 5 minutes or until onion is

Soups & Salads

soft. Drain tomatoes, reserving liquid; chop coarsely and add to vegetables; continue cooking for another 3 minutes. Add beans with their liquid and the tomato liquid plus enough water to total about 3 quarts of soup. Add salt. Bring to boil; simmer 1½ hours. Mash some of the beans if thicker texture is desired; stir in zucchini and remaining seasonings. Cook about 15 minutes or until zucchini is tender. Adjust seasonings.

MARIE'S BOUILLABAISSE

½ pound fresh or frozen haddock fillet, cut up
½ cup celery, diced
½ cup carrots, diced
1 medium potato, diced
1 medium tomato, chopped (optional)
½ bayleaf
½ teaspoon thyme
¼ teaspoon basil
Salt and pepper to taste
1 medium onion, chopped
1 clove garlic, minced
2 tablespoons milk-free margarine
1 small can shrimp, including juice
1 small can clams, including juice
1 small can crab meat, including juice
1 cup sherry or white wine

Combine haddock, potato, celery, carrots, tomato, and seasonings. Add water to barely cover and simmer 15 minutes or until haddock is tender. Meanwhile, saute onion and garlic in the margarine. When haddock is cooked, add sauteed onions and garlic, canned seafood, and wine. Reheat.

Don't let the long list of ingredients discourage you; this goes together in a jiffy. Vary the proportions of fresh, frozen, or canned seafood according to availability and cost.

CLAM CHOWDER

2 tablespoons milk-free margarine
1 small onion, chopped
1 small clove garlic, minced
½ small green pepper, chopped
1 large carrot, diced
1 tomato, peeled and chopped
1 large stalk celery, diced
1 large potato, diced
1 chicken bouillon cube
Dash thyme
1 small bayleaf
1 8-oz. can minced clams (broth included)

Saute onion, garlic, green pepper, and carrot in margarine until onion is golden and slightly tender. Add water to cover; add remaining ingredients except clams. Simmer until vegetables are tender. Add clams and broth. Re-heat.

SWEET 'N SOUR COLESLAW

1 medium head cabbage, shredded
1 medium onion, chopped
1 medium green pepper, chopped
1 tablespoon salt
1 cup vinegar
1 ½ cups sugar
1 teaspoon celery seed
½ teaspoon mustard seed

Combine vegetables and salt in large pan. Cover with boiling water, cover pan and let stand for one hour. Drain well and return to pan. Heat vinegar, sugar and spices until sugar dissolves. Pour over vegetables; mix well. Store in glass container in refrigerator. Let flavors blend for a day before serving. Keeps for several weeks in refrigerator.

TABOOLI

Or, Tabuli, or, Tabbouleh. However you spell it, it makes a great side salad for a buffet or a nutritious extra to have on hand in the refrigerator. (It keeps well for a week.)

¾ cup bulgur (cracked wheat)
1 large tomato, peeled and diced
1 medium onion, chopped
¼ cup fresh parsley, minced
¼ cup fresh mint, minced
6 tablespoons salad or olive oil
3 tablespoons lemon juice
1 teaspoon salt
Dash pepper

Pour boiling water over bulgur in medium size bowl. Cover and let soak half hour or until soft. Drain well. Add tomato, onion, parsley, and mint; mix lightly but well. Combine oil and lemon juice with salt and pepper; shake well to blend. Pour over bulgur and vegetables; mix well. Chill, covered, several hours or overnight. Serve on salad greens, if desired.

CHERRY SALAD

1 17-ounce can sweet dark cherries
1 3-ounce package JELL-O®, any red flavor
1 cup boiling water
2 tablespoons orange juice
¾ cup diced orange sections

Drain cherries, reserving syrup; add cold water to syrup to make 1 cup liquid. Dissolve gelatin in the boiling water; add measured liquid and orange juice. Chill until the consistency of unbeaten egg whites. Fold in cherries and oranges. Pour into a 1-quart mold or individual molds. Chill until firm.

Living...Without Milk

PINEAPPLE AND CARROT SALAD

1 3-oz. package lemon gelatin
1 cup boiling water
1½ cups pineapple juice
1 28-oz. can crushed pineapple, drained
1 cup grated carrots
1 tablespoon vinegar

Dissolve gelatin in boiling water. Add pineapple juice. Cool. Add remaining ingredients; stir. Pour into 1½ quart mold. Chill.

CRANBERRY MOLD

1 3-oz. package JELL-O®, any red flavor
1 cup boiling water
¾ cup 7-Up® or pineapple juice (canned)
1 8-oz. can whole berry cranberry sauce
1 cup diced apples or celery
½ cup coarsely chopped nuts

Dissolve gelatin in boiling water. Add 7-Up or pineapple juice and cranberry sauce. Chill until slightly thickened. Stir in remaining ingredients and pour into 4-cup mold. Chill until firm.

NOTE: Recipe may be doubled; use only 1 cup 7-Up or pineapple juice.

PINEAPPLE-LIME SALAD

1 3-oz. package lime gelatin
¾ cup Tofu "Sour Cream"*
         or: 1 cup thawed Cool Whip®
1 8-oz. can crushed pineapple
½ cup chopped pecans

Drain pineapple, reserving liquid. Make gelatin using liquid plus enough water to make 1¾ cups. Chill until gelatin starts to thicken; fold in remaining ingredients. Pour into 4-cup mold. Chill until firm.

TUNA-MACARONI SALAD

1 cup uncooked elbow macaroni
1 7-ounce can tuna, drained
1 tablespoon grated onion
1 tablespoon minced parsley
¾ cup mayonnaise
½ teaspoon salt
¼ teaspoon pepper
2 tablespoons sweet pickle relish

Cook macaroni according to package directons; drain well and cool. Combine with remaining ingredients. Serve on lettuce.

HAM-RICE SALAD

1⅓ cups Minute® Rice
3 cups diced, cooked ham
1 20-ounce can pineapple chunks, drained
2 cups diced celery
½ cup diced green pepper
1½ cups mayonnaise
1 teaspoon salt
¼ teaspoon pepper
2 tablespoons lemon juice
1 tablespoon grated onion
1 tablespoon prepared mustard

Cook rice according to package directions; cool. Add ham, pineapple, celery, and green pepper; chill. Combine remaining ingredients in separate bowl; chill. Just before serving, toss mixtures together lightly. Serve on lettuce.

SPINACH SALAD

Lots of nutrients here that are missing in the milk-free diet - thiamin, vitamin A, calcium, and iron.

½ pound fresh spinach
1 cup sliced mushrooms (optional)
3 slices bacon, diced
2 teaspoons brown sugar
¼ cup onion, finely chopped
1 ½ tablespoons vinegar
¼ teaspoon salt
1/8 teaspoon dry mustard
Dash paprika

Wash and dry spinach; chill well. When ready to serve, tear into bowl, discarding coarse stems. Cook diced bacon over moderate heat until it starts to brown. Remove all but 2 tablespoons of the bacon fat; add onions; saute until limp but not brown. Add sugar, vinegar, salt, mustard, paprika; bring to boiling. Pour over spinach and mushrooms, if used; toss well until leaves are evenly coated. Serve immediately.

Makes 2 luncheon servings or 4 small salads.

Think of yourself as the Sherlock Holmes of the supermarket and write to the food manufacturer whenever you are uncertain about an ingredient. It will give you the information you need and give the manufacturer an awareness of the importance of not allowing any "hidden" ingredients in his products.

BAKED GOODS

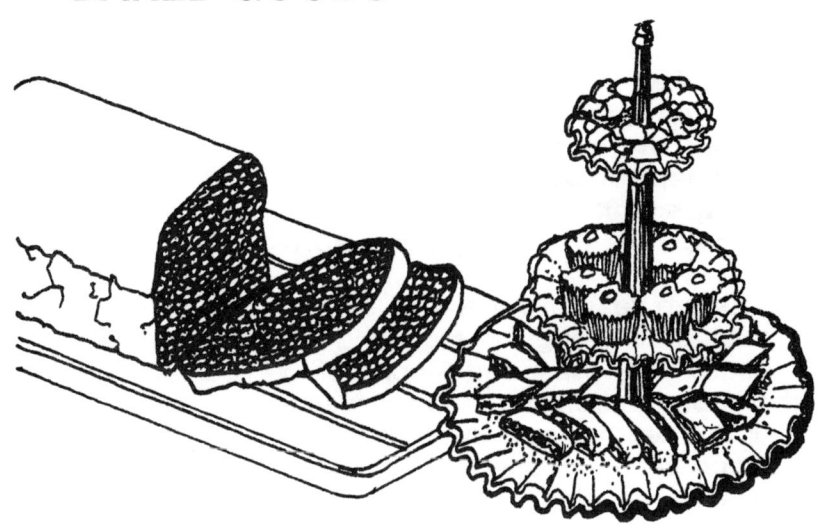

HONEY WHEAT BREAD

The alcohol in the bread cooks out leaving a light, flavorful bread. Make the day ahead for best flavor.

1½ cups all-purpose self-rising flour
1 cup whole wheat flour
1½ teaspoons baking powder
¾ teaspoon salt
3 tablespoons honey
1 bottle (12 ounces) regular beer at room temperature

Sift together dry ingredients. Gently stir in beer and honey; mix just until blended. Turn into greased 9x5x3-inch bread pan.

Bake 50-60 minutes in a 350° oven (or until tester inserted in center comes out clean). Turn out on rack. Cool completely and wrap in foil or plastic.

FEATHER-LITE BREAD

½ cup warm water
2 packages dry yeast
6 eggs, room temperature
¼ cup sugar or honey
½ teaspoon salt
5 cups white flour
½ cup milk-free margarine, soft

Dissolve yeast in water and let stand until it starts to bubble. Beat eggs until light and lemon-colored; add sugar, salt, yeast and 3 cups of the flour. Mix until smooth and elastic. Add margarine and mix again until smooth. Blend in remaining 2 cups flour with wooden spoon to form a soft dough. Cover and let rise until doubled.

Knead dough for 2 minutes on a well-floured surface. Divide dough and shape into two loaves. Place in two well-greased 9x5x3-inch loaf pans. Let rise to top of pans.

Bake 35-40 minutes in a 400° oven.

COFFEE CAN RYE BREAD

1 package active dry yeast
¼ cup lukewarm water
½ cup brown sugar
1 teaspoon salt
1 teaspoon caraway seed
1 tablespoon shortening
2 cups water
3 cups unsifted flour
2 cups light rye flour

Sprinkle active dry yeast over lukewarm water in cup and let stand until dissolved. Measure brown sugar into saucepan and add salt, caraway seed, shortening, and water. Bring to boil, lower heat and simmer gently for five minutes. Let cool to lukewarm and stir in dissolved yeast. Add unsifted flour and beat well. Transfer to greased bowl, cover with damp cloth and place in warm spot until dough has doubled in bulk. Stir down with spoon and blend in rye flour, mixing well. Spoon batter into three greased one pound coffee cans, filling about two-thirds. Place plastic cover over cans and let rise in warm spot until doubled in bulk.

Remove plastic covers. Bake 35 minutes in a 375° oven or until bread tests done when tried with a cake tester. Slide loaves out on rack to cool. Wrap in foil or saran to store.

Makes 3 loaves.

7-UP® BISCUITS

2 cups sifted all-purpose flour
1 teaspoon salt
4 teaspoons baking powder
½ cup shortening
¾ cup 7-Up®
Melted milk-free margarine

Sift dry ingredients into bowl; cut in shortening until mixture resembles coarse corn meal. Add 7-Up all at once; stir briskly with fork until dry ingredients are evenly moistened. Turn onto lightly floured surface; knead quickly 10 times. Roll to ¾" thickness. Allow to rest five minutes. Cut with lightly floured 2-inch cutter. Arrange on baking sheet. Brush lightly with melted margarine.

Bake 10-12 minutes in a 450° oven or until golden brown. Makes 12.

Living...Without Milk

CORN BREAD

1 cup sifted all-purpose flour
1 cup corn meal
¼ cup sugar
2 teaspoons baking powder
½ teaspoon salt
2 eggs
¾ cup water
¼ cup soft milk-free margarine

Sift together dry ingredients into bowl. Add eggs, water, and shortening. Beat just until smooth. Pour into greased 8-inch square pan. Bake 20-25 minutes in a 425° oven.

NOTE: To make handy cakes for your toaster, cut bread into squares and split. Freeze. No need to thaw before toasting.

SCONES

2 cups all-purpose flour
2 tablespoons sugar
2½ teaspoons baking powder
½ teaspoon salt
⅓ cup vegetable shortening
⅓ cup raisins
2 eggs
⅓ cup non-dairy creamer
2 tablespoons sugar

Sift together flour, sugar, baking powder and salt into bowl. Cut in shortening until mixture resembles coarse meal. Add raisins. Break eggs into separate bowl; remove and reserve one tablespoon egg white. Beat remaining eggs; stir in non-dairy creamer. Add all at once to flour and raisin mixture, stirring until flour is moistened. Turn out on lightly floured surface and knead gently 15-20 times. Pat into an 8-inch circle about ½-inch thick; cut into 10 or 12 pie shaped wedges with a floured knife or sharp spatula. Separate wedges. Place on ungreased baking sheet. Beat reserved egg white until foamy; brush over tops. Sprinkle with the remaining 2 tablespoons sugar.

Bake 12-15 minutes in a 425° oven.

BANANA NUT BREAD

2 cups sifted flour
1½ teaspoons baking powder
½ teaspoon baking soda
2-3 bananas (1 cup mashed)
2 eggs
½ cup shortening
1 cup sugar
1½ tablespoons non-dairy creamer
1 teaspoon lemon juice
¼ teaspoon salt
½ cup chopped nuts
½ cup raisins (optional)

MIXER METHOD: Cream together shortening and sugar; add eggs and beat well. Sift together dry ingredients; add to creamed mixture alternately with the combined mashed banana, creamer, and lemon juice. Stir in nuts and raisins. Pour into well-greased 9x5x3-inch or two 8x4x3-inch loaf pans.

BLENDER METHOD: Sift dry ingredients into bowl. Blend bananas to puree; add eggs, shortening, sugar, creamer, lemon juice, and salt; blend until smooth. Pour over dry ingredients; stir just until combined. Stir in nuts and raisins. Pour into well-greased pans.

Bake 9x5x3-inch pan 45 minutes or until done in a 350° oven. Bake 8x4x3-inch pans 40 minutes or until done. Remove from pan; cool on rack.

Living...Without Milk

QUICK APPLESAUCE MUFFINS

1 tablespoon sugar
½ teaspoon cinnamon
1 cup unsifted flour
6 tablespoons sugar
½ teaspoon salt
½ teaspoon baking soda
½ teaspoon cinnamon
½ cup raisins
¼ cup chopped nuts
½ cup applesauce
¼ cup oil
½ teaspoon vanilla
1 egg

Combine the 1 tablespoon sugar and ½ teaspoon cinnamon; set aside. Combine remaining ingredients; blend at low speed 1 minute and beat at medium speed 1 minute. Fill muffin pans ⅔ full. Sprinkle reserved sugar and cinnamon over tops. Bake 15-20 minutes in a 400° oven or until done. Makes 12.

COCONUT KISSES

4 egg whites
½ teaspoon salt
1¼ cups fine granulated sugar
1 teaspoon vanilla
2 cups shredded coconut
24 candied cherries, halved

Beat egg whites and salt until stiff. Gradually add sugar, beating well. Fold in vanilla and coconut. Drop by teaspoonfuls onto ungreased brown paper on cookie sheets. Top with cherries.

Bake 20 minutes in a 350° oven. Slip paper onto wet table. Let stand one minute. Loosen with spatula; remove to racks. Makes four dozen.

Baked Goods

BUTTERSCOTCH OATMEAL COOKIES

1½ cups sifted flour
1 teaspoon baking soda
1 teaspoon salt
1 cup brown sugar
½ cup granulated sugar
1 cup milk-free margarine
2 eggs
1 teaspoon vanilla
3 cups oatmeal

Sift together flour, baking soda, and salt. Add remaining ingredients except oatmeal; beat for two minutes. Blend in oatmeal. Shape into roll or bar (an empty plastic wrap carton makes a good "mold"). Chill overnight. Slice ¼" thick.

Bake 10-12 minutes in a 375° oven. Makes about 3½ dozen.

BANANA ENERGY BARS (BB)

¾ cup soft milk-free margarine
1 cup dark brown sugar, packed
1 egg
½ teaspoon salt
1½ cups mashed ripe bananas
4 cups uncooked regular oats
1 cup raisins
½ cup chopped walnuts

Cream margarine and sugar until light and fluffy. Beat in egg, salt and bananas. Stir in remaining ingredients. Turn into greased 13x9x2-inch baking pan.

Bake 1 hour in 350° oven or until cake tester comes out clean. Cool completely. Cut into 2x1-inch bars.

FROSTED COFFEE COOKIES

½ cup shortening
½ cup brown sugar
½ cup granulated sugar
2 eggs, well beaten
1½ cups flour, sifted
¼ teaspoon salt
½ teaspoon baking soda
½ teaspoon baking powder
½ teaspoon cinnamon
½ teaspoon nutmeg
½ cup cold coffee
½ teaspoon vanilla
½ cup finely chopped nuts
½ cup milk-free margarine
4 cups confectioners' sugar
¼ cup coffee

Cream shortening and sugars until light. Add eggs and beat well. Sift together next six ingredients. Add to first mixture alternately with the ½ cup coffee. Add flavoring and nuts. Spread ¼-inch thick in two well greased 10½x15½-inch shallow pans. Bake 25 minutes in a 350° oven. Combine remaining ingredients, creaming until smooth. Frost cookies while hot and cut into bars when cool.

PEANUT BUTTER SCOTCHIES

½ cup Corn Flake Crumbs
½ teaspoon baking powder
¼ teaspoon salt
½ cup coarsely chopped nuts
¼ cup milk-free margarine
1 cup light brown sugar
⅓ cup peanut butter
2 eggs, slightly beaten
Confectioners' sugar

Combine Corn Flake Crumbs, baking powder, salt, and nuts. Set aside. Melt margarine; remove from heat. Stir in brown sugar and peanut butter until well combined. Add eggs. Beat well. Stir in crumb mixture. Spread in greased 9x9x2-inch baking pan.

Bake 30 minutes in a 350° oven or until tester inserted near center comes out clean. When cool, cut into squares and roll in cofectioners' sugar.

Makes about 25.

BLUEBERRY BARS

½ cup soft milk-free margarine
¼ cup granulated sugar
1 cup sifted flour
½ cup sifted flour
½ teaspoon baking powder
¼ teaspoon salt
1 cup brown sugar, packed
2 eggs, well beaten
½ teaspoon vanilla or almond
½ cup chopped nuts
1 cup fresh blueberries

Mix together first three ingredients until mixture is crumbly. Pat into bottom of greased 9x9-inch square pan. Bake 25 minutes in a 350° oven. Cool.

Meanwhile, sift together next three ingredients. Set aside. With electric mixer, gradually beat brown sugar into eggs; mix in flour mixture just until combined. Stir in flavoring and walnuts. Fold in blueberries gently. Spread evenly over cooled crust. Bake 30 minutes in a 350° oven or until browned and firm to the touch. Cool on rack. Cut into bars. Roll in **confectioners' sugar**, if desired. Makes 2 dozen.

Living...Without Milk

WALNUT BROWNIES

½ cup milk-free margarine
⅓ cup unsweetened cocoa or carob powder
1 teaspoon vanilla
2 eggs
1 cup sugar
¾ cup flour
½ teaspoon baking powder
¼ teaspoon salt
½ cup chopped nuts

Melt margarine; add cocoa or carob powder and vanilla. Cool. Beat together eggs and sugar until thick and lemon-colored. Sift together dry ingredients and stir into cooled cocoa mixture. Stir in nuts. Pour into greased 8-inch square pan.

Bake 25-30 minutes in a 350° oven. Cool in pan; cut into bars.

MAPLE CAKE

2½ cups sifted flour
2 teaspoons baking powder
¾ teaspoon baking soda
½ teaspoon salt
¼ teaspoon ginger
½ cup milk-free margarine
¼ cup sugar
2 eggs
1 cup maple syrup
½ cup hot water

Sift together dry ingredients. Cream together margarine and sugar until light; beat in eggs and syrup until well blended. Add dry ingredients alternately with hot water blending in at low mixer speed. Pour into 2 greased, lined 8-inch round pans.

Bake 30-35 minutes in a 350° oven. Cool completely on racks before removing from pans. Frost.

NOTE: To bake as **CUPCAKES** fill paper baking cups in muffin pans half full. Makes 18. Bake 20 minutes.

MAPLE FROSTING

6 tablespoons milk-free margarine
1 teaspoon vanilla
3 cups confectioners' sugar
Dash salt
½ cup maple syrup

Combine all ingredients in mixer bowl and beat until mixture is of good spreading consistency. If necessary, thin with non-dairy creamer or coffee.

CHOCOLATE MAYONNAISE CAKE

2 cups unsifted all-purpose flour
1 cup sugar
½ cup unsweetened cocoa or carob powder
1½ teaspoons baking powder
1 teaspoon baking soda
1 cup whole-egg mayonnaise
1 cup cold water
1 teaspoon vanilla

Sift together dry ingredients. Stir in mayonnaise. Gradually stir in water and vanilla until smooth. Pour into two greased and lined 8-inch layer pans.

Bake 30 minutes in a 350° oven or until cake tests done. Cool completely before removing from pans.

NOTE: May also be baked in one 8x12x2-inch or one 9x9x2-inch pan. No need to line pan; just cool and frost in pan.

Living...Without Milk

FRUIT COCKTAIL CAKE

1¼ cups flour
1 cup sugar
1 teaspoon baking soda
1 16-ounce can fruit cocktail, undrained
1 egg, slightly beaten
1 cup brown sugar
1 cup nuts, chopped
1 teaspoon cinnamon

Combine flour, sugar, and baking soda. Add fruit cocktail and egg; mix well. Pour into greased 9x13-inch pan. Combine brown sugar, nuts, and cinnamon; sprinkle over top.

Bake 45 minutes in a 325° oven. Serve warm or cold with milk-free whipped topping.

NOTE: For 6x10-inch pan, halve all ingredients except egg. Bake 35 minutes.

JOSHUA'S APPLE CAKE

2 tablespoons milk-free margarine
1 cup sugar
1 egg
3 cups pared, diced apples
½ cup chopped nuts
1 teaspoon vanilla
1 cup flour
¼ teaspoon salt
¼ teaspoon cinnamon
1 teaspoon baking soda

Cream together margarine, sugar, and egg. Stir in apples, nuts, and vanilla. Combine remaining dry ingredients and add to apple mixture; mix well. Turn into greased, floured 9x5x3-inch pan.

Bake 50-60 minutes in a 350º oven. Cool 15 minutes before removing from pan. Serve warm with non-dairy whipped topping or GOLDEN SAUCE*.

SARAH'S SPICE CAKE

1 ½ cups sifted cake flour
2 teaspoons baking powder
½ teaspoon salt
½ teaspoon each: cinnamon, cloves, nutmeg, allspice
⅓ cup shortening
⅔ cup Squash Milk*
1 large egg
1 cup sugar

Sift together dry ingredients into bowl. Place remaining ingredients in blender in order listed; blend until smooth. Pour blended mixture gradually into sifted flour mixture; stir lightly until just smooth. Pour into greased and floured 8-inch square pan.

Bake 35 minutes in a 350º oven. Cool in pan. Serve with GOLDEN SAUCE*.

GOLDEN SAUCE

1 egg
4 tablespoons soft milk-free margarine
1 teaspoon vanilla
1 cup confectioners' sugar

Place ingredients in blender in order listed. Blend until smooth. Refrigerate if not serving shortly.

Living...Without Milk

COCONUT BIRTHDAY CAKE

Looks and tastes like a conventional birthday cake but without the milk. Make the day before for best flavor.

½ cup milk-free margarine
1 cup sugar
3 eggs
2 cups sifted cake flour
2½ teaspoons baking powder
½ teaspoon salt
½ cup bottled Coconut Milk beverage
1 teaspoon orange flavoring

Cream the margarine and gradually add sugar. Cream together until light and fluffy. Beat in eggs one at a time, beating well after each addition. Sift together cake flour, baking powder, and salt. Combine coconut milk and orange flavoring and add alternately with dry ingredients beginning and ending with flour mixture. Pour into 2 8-inch wax paper lined cake pans.

Bake 20-25 minutes in a 375° oven. Remove from pan; cool completely before filling and frosting.

COCONUT FILLING

⅓ cup sugar
1½ tablespoons cornstarch
¼ teaspoon salt
1 cup bottled Coconut Milk beverage
2 egg yolks, slightly beaten
1 tablespoon milk-free margarine
1 teaspoon orange flavoring

Combine sugar, cornstarch, and salt in saucepan. Gradually add coconut milk; blend well. Cook over medium heat, stirring constantly until mixture boils and thickens. Blend a bit of the hot mixture into the egg yolks; return to hot mixture in saucepan and cook until mixture bubbles, stirring constantly. Stir in margarine and flavoring. Cool.

FLUFFY FROSTING

2 egg whites
1 cup sugar
1/8 teaspoon cream of tartar
¼ cup water
1 teaspoon vanilla

Combine ingredients except vanilla in top of double boiler. Place over boiling water and beat with rotary beater or portable mixer until mixture holds its shape (about 7 minutes). Fold in vanilla.

BANANA SPICE CUPCAKES

¼ cup soft milk-free margarine
⅔ cup sugar
1 egg
1 cup flour
1 teaspoon baking powder
½ teaspoon salt
½ teaspoon baking soda
¼ teaspoon cinnamon
¼ teaspoon nutmeg
¼ teaspoon allspice
½ cup mashed ripe banana
1 tablespoon non-dairy creamer
1 tablespoon water

Cream together margarine and sugar; add egg and beat until well blended. Sift together dry ingredients and spices. Combine banana, creamer, and water. Add dry ingredients to creamed mixture alternately with banana mixture and mix well. Fill paper baking cups in muffin pans half full.

Bake 20-25 minutes in a 375° oven. Makes 12.

Living...Without Milk

WHOLE WHEAT MAPLE CAKE

A very easy recipe. Good for breakfast or brown bag lunches.

1 cup maple syrup
½ cup salad oil or melted milk-free margarine
1 teaspoon each cloves, nutmeg, cinnamon, salt
1 cup seedless raisins
1 cup cold water
1¾ cups whole wheat flour
¼ cup cornstarch
1 teaspoon baking soda
½ cup chopped nuts

Place syrup, oil, spices, raisins, and water in saucepan. Bring to boil and boil for 4 minutes. Chill thoroughly. Sift together the whole wheat flour, cornstarch, and baking soda three times. Add to the boiled mixture along with the nuts. Beat well. Pour into greased 9x5x3-inch pan.

Bake 60 minutes in a 350° oven.

NOTE: 2 cups all-purpose flour may be substituted for the whole wheat flour and cornstarch. Sift only once with the baking soda.

COFFEE RICH POUND CAKE (R)

1½ cups sugar
¾ cup hydrogenated shortening
6 eggs
3¼ cups sifted cake flour
1 tablespoon double action baking powder
1 teaspoon salt
¾ cup Coffee Rich®
1 teaspoon vanilla
½ teaspoon butter flavoring

Cream together sugar and shortening until light and fluffy. Beat in eggs, one at a time. Sift together cake flour, baking powder, and salt.

Combine Coffee Rich®, vanilla, and butter flavoring and add alternately with dry ingredients, beginning and ending with flour mixture. Pour into 3 9-inch wax paper lined or greased and floured cake pans.

Bake in 350° oven 25 minutes or until cake pulls away from sides of pan. Remove from pan. Cool. Frost as desired.

MOIST ORANGE CAKE

1 cup milk-free margarine
1 orange
5 eggs, separated
1 cup sugar
1 cup flour
3½ teaspoons baking powder
2 cups water
1 cup sugar
1 tablespoon orange curacao

Melt margarine and set aside to cool. Grate rind from orange and extract juice (exact amount is not important). Combine egg yolks and the 1 cup sugar and beat well. Stir in melted margarine, rind, juice, flour, and baking powder. Beat egg whites until stiff and carefully fold into batter. Pour into greased 8x10-inch or 9x9-inch pan.

Bake 10 minutes in a 375° oven; reduce temperature to 350° and bake 30 minutes longer. Cool 15 minutes.

Meanwhile, combine the water and remaining sugar; boil 10 minutes. Add flavoring; pour hot syrup over cooled cake. (Flavor is best the second day.)

Living...Without Milk

COCONUT ORANGE CUSTARD PIE

3 eggs
¾ cup sugar
½ cup water
½ cup orange juice (preferably fresh)
2 tablespoons flour
Dash salt
½ cup shredded coconut
1 teaspoon grated orange rind
1 8-inch unbaked pie shell

Beat eggs well; gradually add sugar. Beat in the remaining ingredients except coconut. Pour mixture into pie shell; sprinkle coconut on top. Bake 20 minutes in a 425° oven. Reduce temperature to 350° and bake 10 minutes longer or until knife inserted halfway between center and edge comes out clean.

PUMPKIN PIE

1½ cups canned pumpkin
½ cup brown sugar
½ cup granulated sugar
1¼ cups Squash "Milk"*
1 tablespoon flour
3 tablespoons milk-free margarine, melted
3 eggs
½ teaspoon salt
1 teaspoon cinnamon
¼ teaspoon each nutmeg and cloves
1 9-inch unbaked pie shell

Place ingredients in blender in order listed and blend until smooth. (Or, place in bowl and beat with rotary beater until smooth.) Pour into pie shell.
Bake 15 minutes in a 425° oven. Reduce temperature to 350° and bake another 45 minutes or until knife inserted halfway between center and edge comes out clean. Cool.

Baked Goods

STRAWBERRY ANGEL PIE

3 egg whites
1 teaspoon vanilla
¼ teaspoon cream of tartar
Dash salt
1 cup sugar
1 10-ounce package frozen strawberries
1 3-ounce package strawberry gelatin
1¼ cups boiling water
1 4½-ounce container Cool Whip®

Combine egg whites, vanilla, cream of tartar, and salt; beat until frothy. Gradually add sugar, beating until very stiff peaks form and sugar is dissolved. Spoon into lightly greased 9-inch pie plate and shape into shell, swirling sides high. Bake 1 hour in a 275º oven. Turn off heat and let dry in oven with the door closed for at least two hours (or overnight).

Meanwhile, thaw strawberries; drain. Dissolve gelatin in boiling water; chill until mixture is the consistency of unbeaten egg white. Fold in thawed strawberries and Cool Whip® . Chill until mixture mounds slightly when spooned. Pile into meringue shell. Chill until firm.

BLUEBERRY TARTS

1½ tablespoons cornstarch
½ cup sugar
½ cup water
3 cups blueberries
1 tablespoon milk-free margarine
6 baked tart shells

Combine cornstarch, sugar, and water. Add washed blueberries and margarine. Cook and stir over medium heat until mixture is thickened and clear. Cool slightly. Fill tart shells with mixture. To serve, top with milk-free whipped topping.

Living...Without Milk

DREAM PUFFS

Pure "junk food" - but we all have our weak days.

1 cup water
½ cup milk-free margarine
1 cup all-purpose flour
¼ teaspoon salt
4 eggs

Bring water, butter, and salt to a rolling boil in saucepan. Add flour; stir vigorously over low heat until mixture leaves sides of the pan and forms a ball. Cool slightly. Add eggs, one at a time, beating until smooth after each addition. Mixture will be stiff. Drop by large spoonfuls about 3 inches apart on ungreased cookie sheet. (Recipe makes 12 large puffs but smaller ones may be made.)

Bake 35-40 minutes in a 400° oven, until puffed and brown. Turn off heat and open door; allow to remain in oven an additional 20 minutes. Slice off tops; reserve. Remove any filaments of soft dough inside; cool.

FILLING

½ cup milk-free margarine
½ cup white vegetable shortening
1 cup granulated sugar
3 tablespoons flour
⅔ cup non-dairy creamer
1½ teaspoons vanilla

To prepare filling, combine margarine, shortening, and sugar; cream at high speed for 3 minutes or until very creamy and sugar is dissolved. Add flour, one tablespoon at a time, then creamer and vanilla. Beat, scraping bowl and beaters several times, for 10-15 minutes or until very fluffy. Use to fill cooled puffs. Dust with confectioners' sugar, if desired.

HAPPY ENDINGS

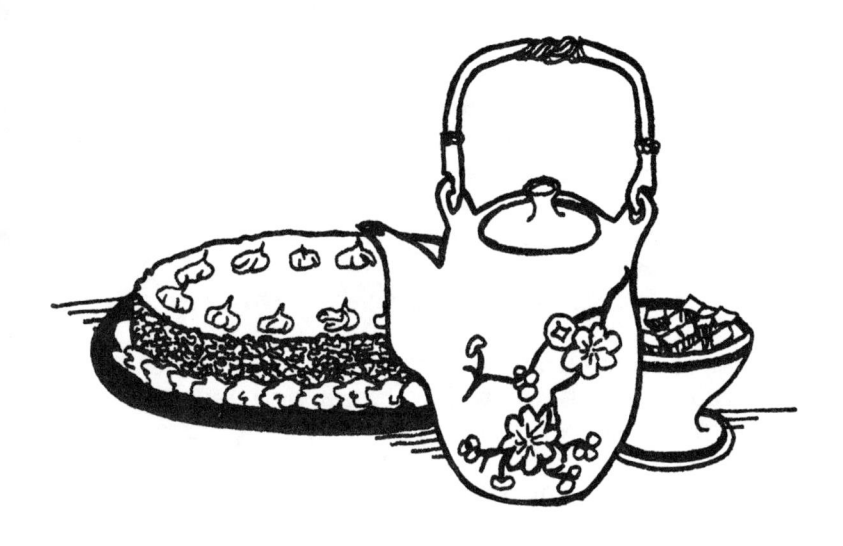

RUM MOUSSE

1 package milk-free lady fingers
3 eggs, separated
½ cup sugar
1 9-ounce container Cool Whip®
1 teaspoon vanilla
2 tablespoons light rum

Wash and dry eggs well before separating; bring to room temperature. Arrange lady fingers in bottom of 8x8x2 pan. Beat egg yolks adding sugar slowly and beating until thick and lemon colored. Beat egg whites until stiff. Fold yolks into whites, then fold in Cool Whip®. Add flavorings and pour mixture over lady fingers. Sprinkle with shaved unsweetened chocolate, if desired.

Freeze 4 hours or more but remove from freezer a few minutes before serving.

CHEESELESS CHEESECAKE

1 ¼ cups graham cracker crumbs
¼ cup milk-free margarine, melted
1 tablespoon sugar
½ teaspoon cinnamon
½ cup boiling water
1 1-oz. package lemon gelatin
2 tablespoons lemon juice
½ teaspoon grated lemon rind
2 cups crumbled tofu
1 10-oz. container dessert whip, thawed

Press excess moisture from tofu; crumble and measure. Place on paper towel and let any additional moisture drain while preparing remaining ingredients. Combine crumbs, margarine, sugar, and cinnamon and press onto bottom of 8" round spring form pan or cake pan. Set aside. Pour boiling water into blender container, add gelatin and blend until dissolved. Add lemon juice, rind, and part of the tofu. Blend until smooth. Add remaining tofu gradually; continue to blend until smooth. Pour into large bowl. Add dessert whip and combine with spatula or mixer at low speed. Pour over crust. Chill until set. For a special treat, serve with sweetened fresh or frozen strawberries.

NOTE: If you prefer not to use frozen dessert whip, you may add ¼ cup non-dairy liquid creamer to the blended ingredients and substitute a meringue made of four egg whites, stiffly beaten with ½ cup sugar and ½ teaspoon vanilla, for the dessert whip. This will make a lighter, less rich cheesecake.

TWIST O'LEMON

1 envelope unflavored gelatin
½ cup boiling water
1 lemon
½ cup sugar
Dash salt
2 eggs
½ cup non-dairy creamer
1 cup ice cubes (about 5)

Remove about ⅔ of the peel from the lemon in thin strips. Squeeze 2 tablespoons juice from the lemon and set aside. Put gelatin and boiling water in blender; cover and blend on low until gelatin is dissolved. Add two ice cubes and lemon peel; blend to grate. Add sugar, lemon juice, salt, eggs, and creamer. Blend on high speed adding ice cubes, one at a time, until ice is melted. Pour into serving bowl or dishes. Chill.

NOTE: Extra good with a topping of sliced, slightly sweetened fresh strawberries.

GRANOLA APPLE CRISP

1 cup Granola*
½ cup flour
1 cup sugar
1 teaspoon cinnamon
½ cup milk-free margarine
4 cups sliced apples, pared

Rub together flour, sugar, cinnamon, and margarine; mix in Granola. Place apples in greased 8x8x2-inch baking dish. Drop Granola mixture over apples by spoonfuls. Bake 40 minutes in a 350° oven.

ORANGE VELVET SHERBET (R)

1 quart Coffee Rich®
½ cup lemon juice
3½ cups orange juice (1-6 oz. can frozen orange juice reconstituted)
3 cups sugar
1 tablespoon unflavored gelatin
¼ cup cold water

Blend together Coffee Rich®, citrus juices, and sugar until sugar is dissolved. Dissolve gelatin in cold water; melt over hot water bath. Beating, add to Coffee Rich® mixture until well blended.

Freeze until firm using 8 parts ice to 1 part salt.

PHILADELPHIA ICE CREAM (R)

1 quart Coffee Rich®
¾ cup sugar
1 teaspoon vanilla
1 pinch salt

Mix all ingredients to dissolve sugar. Freeze until firm using 8 parts ice to 1 part salt.

NOTE: For COFFEE ICE CREAM, dissolve 1½ tablespoons instant coffee in 2 tablespoons hot water and add to ice cream mixture. For MAPLE NUT ICE CREAM, add 1 cup finely chopped nuts and substitute maple flavoring for vanilla in ice cream mix. For PEPPERMINT STICK ICE CREAM, substitute ½ pound crushed peppermint stick candy for sugar and vanilla.

NOTE: These recipes freeze equally well in the in-freezer electric ice cream maker using only 24 ounces of the mixture for each batch.

BUTTERSCOTCH SWIRL ICE CREAM

¼ cup brown sugar
2 tablespoons milk-free margarine
2 tablespoons dark corn syrup
3 tablespoons non-dairy creamer

Combine all ingredients; boil 2 minutes. Cool. Fold into 1 pint vanilla PHILADELPHIA ICE CREAM* for marbled effect. Freeze.

NEW ENGLAND CRANBERRY-BANANA SHRUB (BB)

2 cups cranberry juice cocktail
3 ripe bananas
1½ cups orange juice
1 tablespoon lemon juice

In an ice cube tray freeze cranberry juice. In electric blender container combine bananas, orange juice and lemon juice. Cover and process until smooth. Add frozen cranberry juice. Cover and process until melted.

JEWELLED BAVARIAN CREAM

1 3-oz. package Jell-O® , any red flavor
1 cup boiling water
½ cup non-dairy creamer

Dissolve gelatin in boiling water. Combine ½ cup of the gelatin mixture with the ½ cup non-dairy creamer. Chill in small mixing bowl. Add cold water to remaining gelatin to make 1¼ cups. Pour into 8" square pan and chill until very firm. Beat creamy portion with mixer until fluffy. Dice clear portion into small cubes and fold into the cream. Spoon into serving dishes and chill.

Living...Without Milk

ORANGE-PINEAPPLE TAPIOCA

½ cup sugar
3 tablespoons tapioca
¼ teaspoon salt
1¾ cups orange juice (about)
2 tablespoons milk-free margarine
1 egg yolk
1 egg white
2 tablespoons sugar
1 8-oz. can crushed pineapple
½ teaspoon grated lemon rind

Drain pineapple, reserving liquid. Add enough orange juice to make 2 cups. Combine sugar, tapioca, salt, and egg yolk in pan. Add juices and margarine; let stand 5 minutes. Cook and stir over medium heat until mixture comes to a boil; stir in lemon rind. Beat egg white with the 2 tablespoons of sugar until peaks form. Gradually add hot mixture to beaten white, stirring quickly just until blended. Fold in pineapple. Cool 20 minutes. Stir. Chill.

PINA COLADA TAPIOCA

3 tablespoons tapioca
2 tablespoons sugar
Dash salt
2 cups Pina Colada
1 egg, separated
2 tablespoons sugar
½ teaspoon vanilla
½ teaspoon almond flavor

Mix tapioca, salt, 2 tablespoons sugar, Pina Colada, and yolk in saucepan. Let stand 5 minutes. Beat egg white until foamy; gradually beat in remaining 2 tablespoons sugar, beating to soft peaks. Set aside. Cook tapioca mixture over medium heat to a full boil, stirring constantly - 6 to 8 minutes. Gradually add to beaten white, stirring quickly just until blended. Stir in vanilla and almond flavoring. Cool 20 minutes. Stir. Chill.

STRAWBERRY TOFU POPSICLES

A good way to introduce tofu to the younger set ... creamy and delicious with only a slight hint of soy flavor.

1 envelope unflavored gelatin
½ cup sugar
½ cup boiling water
1 cup whole frozen strawberries
1 cup tofu, crumbled and drained

Combine gelatin, sugar, and boiling water in blender; blend on high until gelatin is dissolved. Remove center cap from lid and add strawberries, one at a time; blend until smooth. Add tofu; blend on low speed just until mixture is smooth. Fill popsicle molds or small paper cups; insert sticks and freeze.

KRACKLE KORN

1 cup maple syrup
1 tablespoon milk-free margarine
2 tablespoons water
2 quarts popped corn
1 cup nuts, optional

Boil syrup, water, and margarine in saucepan until mixture reaches 275° on candy thermometer (or forms a hard ball). Pour quickly over popped corn and nuts, stirring constantly.

NOTE: Puffed wheat makes a good substitute for the popped corn. Raisins make a flavorful, nutritious addition.

Living...Without Milk

8-MINUTE CHOCOLATE FUDGE

2 cups granulated sugar
2 squares unsweetened chocolate
Dash salt
¼ cup water
¼ cup non-dairy creamer
2 tablespoons milk-free margarine
1 teaspoon vanilla
½ cup walnuts, chopped (optional)

Combine sugar, chocolate, salt, water and creamer in saucepan and place over HIGH heat. Bring to boil; lower to MEDIUM heat. Boil stirring occasionally until ingredients are blended. This should take four minutes at the most; color will look more even. Remove from heat; immediately add margarine and vanilla. Beat with mixer until batter starts to thicken; quickly add nuts and pour into shallow, greased 5x9-inch pan. Cool.

EASY PENUCHE

1 pound brown sugar (2⅓ cups)
½ cup non-dairy creamer
¼ cup water
2 tablespoons milk-free margarine
1 teaspoon vanilla
½ cup walnuts, chopped

Combine brown sugar, creamer, and water; stir well to break up any lumps of sugar. Cook as directed above except allow to cool five minutes before beating and use shallow 8x8-inch pan. Mark in squares before completely cool.

NOTE: Once you get the "feel" of these recipes, you'll be able to satisfy sweet tooth cravings with fudge that rivals the candy thermometer, kneaded kind.

PRODUCT INFORMATION DIRECTORY

Manufacturers are anxious to provide you with the information you need to make your diet planning easier. Do not hesitate to write when you need to know more about the ingredients in a product. Many of them have current lists of their milk-free products available and most of them will respond cordially to your questions. Because products are constantly being re-formulated, the lists are updated frequently; the safest thing to do is to contact these manufacturers directly for the latest lists.

I have included a representative sampling of some milk-free products that are likely to remain so in the near future but your best protection is to check the label each time you purchase a product.

BEST FOODS DIV. OF CPC INTERNATIONAL, Consumer Services Dept., International Plaza, Englewood Cliffs, NJ 17632

Holiday margarine, Mazola Diet imitation margarine, Mazola margarine (unsalted variety only), Nucoa margarine, Nucoa soft margarine.

BEATRICE FOODS CO., Two North LaSalle St., Chicago, IL 60602.

Shedd's Willow Run Soy Bean Margarine (available in health food stores)

BORDEN, INC., Customer Service, 180 East Broad St., Columbus, OH 43215.

CAMPBELL SOUP CO., General Offices, Camden, NJ 08101

FEARN SOYA FOODS, 4520 James Place, Melrose Park, IL 60160.

Fearn Soya Powder and Granules, Soy/o mixes.

Living...Without Milk

GENERAL FOODS CONSUMER CENTER, Nutrition Services, 250 North St., White Plains, NY 10625.

Send for their list of milk-free products and the leaflet, "Special Recipes and Allergy Aids".

GENERAL MILLS CONSUMER SERVICE, 9200 Wayzata Blvd., P.O. Box 1113, Minneapolis, MN 55440.

GERBER PRODUCTS COMPANY, Professional Communications Dept., 445 State St., Fremont, MI 49412.

Ask for "Ingredients: Gerber Baby Foods". It is an invaluable guide for mothers of babies with food allergies; lists nutrients, additives, and ingredients in Gerber baby food products.

H.J. HEINZ CO., Home Economics Dept., P.O. Box 57, Pittsburgh, PA 15230.

HERSHEY CHOCOLATE COMPANY, 19 East Chocolate Avenue, Hershey, PA 17033.

For those who are not also allergic to chocolate, both Hershey's Baking Chocolate (bitter) and Hershey's Cocoa are derived exclusively from the cocoa bean, are unsweetened, and contain no other ingredients.

HUDSON PHARMACEUTICAL CORPORATION, 21 Henderson Drive, West Caldwell, NJ 07006.

Many of their vitamins and over-the-counter drugs are lactose-free; inquire about your specific interests.

ITT CONTINENTAL BAKING COMPANY, INC., P.O. Box 731, Halstead Ave., Rye, NY 10580.

Fresh Horizons (white bread only), Family Rye Bread, Beefsteak Soft Rye Bread, Beefsteak Hearty Rye Bread.

Product Information Directory

KEEBLER COMPANY, 677 Larch Ave., Elmhurst, IL 60126.

LEDERLE LABS, Product Information, Middletown Rd., Pearl River, NY 10965.

LIBBY, McNEILL & LIBBY, INC., Home Economics Dept., 200 South Michigan Ave., Chicago, IL 60604

MALABAR FORMULAS, 9080 Bloomfield St., #203, Cypress, CA 90630.

Malabar Milk Digestant tablets.

MITCHELL FOODS, Fredonia, NY 14063.

Perx and Polyperx

NABISCO, INC., Consumer Services, East Hanover, NJ 07936.

They will send you a current list of their cookies, crackers, cereals, and mixes that do not contain milk or milk derivatives.

PFIZER PHARMACEUTICALS, PFIZER, INC., 235 E. 42nd St., New York, NY 10017.

THE PILLSBURY COMPANY, Consumer Affairs, Box 550, Minneapolis, MN 55440.

Because formulas change from time to time, they prefer to send you their latest list. Mention your specific allergy or product interest.

PROCTOR & GAMBLE, Box 599, Cincinnati, OH 45201.

QUAKER OATS CO., Consumer Services, Chicago, IL 60654.

RALSTON PURINA COMPANY, Office of Consumer Affairs, Checkerboard Square, St. Louis, MO 63188.

RICH PRODUCTS CORPORATION, P.O. Box 245, 1145 Niagara St., Buffalo, NY 14240.

Coffee Rich, Poly Rich, Rich's Whip Topping, Rich Whip

A.H. ROBINS COMPANY, Office of Medical Research, 1211 Sherwood Ave., Richmond, VA 23220.

SCHIFF BIO-FOOD PRODUCTS, Moonachie Ave., Moonachie, NJ 07074.

Lactozyme milk digestant tablets, Time Release Single Day vitamins and other vitamin preparations suitable for milk-free diets.

SOVEX NATURAL FOODS, INC., Box 310, Collegedale, TN 37315

Good Shepherd Traditional cereal, Sovex Honey Almond, Crunchy, and Fruit & Nut cereals, Prothin snack chips.

SUGARLO COMPANY, 600 Fire Rd., P.O. Box 1100, Pleasantville, NJ 08232.

LactAid® lactase enzyme

MAIL ORDER SOURCES OF MILK-FREE FOODS

CHICAGO DIETETIC SUPPLY, INC., 405 E. Shawmut Ave., La Grange, IL 60525.

ENER-G FOODS, INC., P.O. Box 24723, Seattle, WA 98124

WALNUT ACRES NATURAL FOODS, Penns Creek, PA 17862

OTHER SOURCES OF HELP

ALLERGY INFORMATION ASSOCIATION, Room 7, 25 Poynter Drive, Weston, Ontario, M9R 1K8, Canada

The purpose of AIA is to enable and encourage members to stay well by learning all about their allergy or sensitivity. Ask about their current membership rate which includes an "Information Kit" and four quarterly newsletters.

AMERICAN ALLERGY ASSOCIATION, P.O. Box 640, Menlo Park, CA 94025

Send for their list of available pamphlets.

AMERICAN DIGESTIVE DISEASE SOCIETY, 420 Lexington Ave., New York, NY 10017

Free pamphlets are available on various digestive disorders. Members receive a health news letter and personal counseling or a doctor referral.

ASTHMA AND ALLERGY FOUNDATION OF AMERICA, 19 W. 44th St., New York, NY 10036

Ask for a sample copy of their newsletter, "In Touch" and a list of their available pamphlets. Membership is also available.

NATIONAL INSTITUTE OF ALLERGY AND INFECTIOUS DISEASES, National Institutes of Health, Bethesda, MD 20205

For more information about "Food Allergy", send for their free pamphlet #75-533.

Have you read any good labels lately?

GENERAL INDEX

A
Addresses; food and drug manufacturers, **127**
Addresses; sources of help, **131**
Alcohol; effect on lactose intolerance, **16**
Allergy Information Association (Canada), 131
Allergy to milk, **11-15**
Alternative food sources of vitamins and nutrients, **27**
American Allergy Association, 131
American Digestive Disease Society, 131
Annand, Dr. J.; milk's relation to heart disease, **11**
Asthma and Allergy Foundation of America, 131

B
Banana Bunch, Ackn. **36**
Bananas; nutritional and medical benefits, **26**
Best Foods, Ackn. **36**
Blood test to determine lactose intolerance, **13**
Breath-hydrogen test to determine lactose intolerance, **14**
Butter substitute, **33**

C
Cheese substitute, **33**
Chocolate substitute, **33**
Chemicals (natural) in milk, **14**
Coconut milk, **34**

Convenience food substitutes, **37**
Cream substitute, **33**

D
Depression; a symptom of lactose intolerance, **11**
Diagnosis of lactose intolerance, **13**
Diarrhea; frequent symptom of lactose intolerance, **11**
Diet chart (pull-out), **23-24**
Digestion of milk; making it easier, **29**

E
Ethnic groups; incidence of lactose intolerance, **16**

F
Foods to avoid on a milk-free diet, **18-19**

G
Galactose, **29**
Galactosemia, **29**
Gastroenteritis and lactose intolerance, **16**
Glucose, **29**

H
Help for milk-free diets, **33**
Hidden ingredients; milk additives in non-dairy products, **14-15**
Hyperactivity; symptom of lactose intolerance, **11**

I
Iron, other sources of, **28**
Irritable Bowel Syndrome (IBS), **15**

L
Lactaid, 29
Lactase enzyme, 13
Lactase tablets, 30
Lactobacillus acidophilus, 30
Lactose (milk sugar), 13
Lactose intolerance; 11-17
    blood test, 13
    breath-hydrogen test, 14
    definition, 15-17
    in adults, 14
    in children, 14
    incidence, 11
    incidence in ethnic groups, 16
Levine, Dr. M; lactose intolerance in children, 13

M
Mail order sources of milk-free food, 130
Mandell, Dr. M.; milk allergy, 12
Medicines, lactose in, 21
Milk additives in foods, 19
Milk allergy, 11-15
Milk allergy and arthritis, 12-13
Milk allergy and ulcers, 11
Milk digestant tablets, 30
Milk products, 14
Milk sensitivity; inherited, 14
Milk substitutes; coconut milk, 34
    creamer, non-dairy 34
    soy, 35
    squash, 35
Mono-sodium-glutamate (MSG), 20

N
National Institute of Allergy and Infectious Diseases, 131
Nervous system, impact of milk on, 12
Non-dairy creamers, 34
Nutrition on a milk-free diet, 25-28
"Nutrition Labeling - Tools for its use", 26

O
Oster, Dr. K.; milk's relation to heart disease, 11

P
Paige, Dr. David, 25
Philpott, Dr. W.H.; milk and emotionally disturbed patients, 12
Physician's (your) recommendations, 22
Potassium; sources of and need for, 25-28
Product information, 127
Products to check carefully, 20

R
Randolph, Dr. T.; milk and rheumatoid arthritis, 12
Recipes, adjusting, 48
Riboflavin; other sources of, 27
Rich Products Corp., Ackn 36

S
Sataline, Dr. Lee; lactose intolerance, 15-17
Seed and nut "milks", 35
Sources of help and information, 131
Soy milk substitutes, 35
Speer, Dr. Frederick; milk allergy, 32
Squash "milk", 35

Standard recipes, 33
Sublingual test 12
"Sweet Acidophilus" milk,, 30
Symptoms of milk sensitivity, 11

T
Thiamine, other sources of, 27
Tofu; soy cheese, 31-32
Trumbull, Dr. J.A.; milk allergy and rheumatoid arthritis, 12

U
Ulcers, 12

V
Vitamins A and C, other sources of, 27-28

W
Whey; an ingredient of milk 14

X
Xanthine oxidase; 11
X-rays; avoidance of 17

RECIPE INDEX

A
Antipasto tray, 61
Appetizers and Dips,
  Antipasto Tray, 61
  Baked Clams Oregano, 58
  Cocktail Meatballs, 58
  Cocktail Mix, 59
  Dieter's Delite Nibblers, 62
  Marinated Artichokes, 60
  Seafood Remoulade, 57
  Spicy Marinated Mushrooms, 60
  Tangy Vegetable Dip, 62
  Tofu Dip, 61
Apple Cake, Joshua's, 110
Apple Crisp, Granola, 121
Artichokes, Marinated, 60

B
Banana Energy Bars, 105
Banana Hula 50
Banana Nut Bread 103
Banana Shrub, New England Cranberry 123
Banana Spice Cupcakes 113
Bavarian Cream, Jewelled 123
Bean Casserole, Baked 86
Bean Pot Soup 90
Beans, Vegetarian Baked 85

Beef and Vegetable casserole, 66
Beef 'n Pepper Steak, 64
Beef Ragout, Oven, 66
Beef Batter for deep frying, 40
Beverages
  Banana Hula, 50
  Berry Tasty Shake, 51
  Creamy "Shake", 50
  Fresh Fruit Smoothy, 51
  Golden Eggnog, 51
Biscuits, 7-Up 101
Blueberry Bars, 107
Blueberry Tarts, 117
Bouillabaisse, Marie's, 93
Bread Crumbs, seasoned, 43
Breads and Muffins
  Banana Nut Bread, 103
  Coffee Can Rye Bread, 100
  Corn Bread, 102
  Cranberry Nut Muffins, 52
  Feather-Lite Bread, 100
  Honey Wheat Bread, 99
  Orange Crumb Coffee Cake, 53
  Pancakes, 56
  Quick Applesauce Muffins, 104
  Scones, 102

7-Up Biscuits, **101**
Breakfast Cookies, **52**
Brownies, Walnut, **108**
Butterscotch Oatmeal
   Cookies, **105**
Butterscotch Swirl Ice
   Cream **123**

C
Cakes
   Banana Spice Cupcakes, **113**
   Chocolate Mayonnaise
      Cake, **109**
   Coconut Birthday Cake, **112**
   Coffee Rich Pound
      Cake, **114**
   Fruit Cocktail Cake, **110**
   Joshua's Apple Cake, **110**
   Maple Cake, **108**
   Moist Orange cake, **115**
   Sarah's Spice Cake, **111**
   Whole Wheat Maple
      Cake, **114**
Carrots, Baked, **87**
Celery Soup, Cream of, **91**
Cereal, Cold, **54**
Cheesecake, Cheeseless, **120**
Cherry Salad, **95**
Chick-a-Bobs, **70**
Chicken
   Baked Stuffed Chicken
      Breasts, **73**
   Chick-a-Bobs, **70**
   Chicken Macaroni
      Casserole, **70**
   Chicken Normandy, **72**
   Oven Barbecued
      Chicken, **68**
   Pot Roasted Chicken, **72**
   Skillet Herb Chicken, **68**
   Sweet and Sour
      Chicken, **71**
   Versatile Baked
      Chicken, **69**
Chili con Carne, **80**
Chocolate Fudge, 8-
   Minute, **126**
Chocolate Mayonnaise
   Cake, **109**
"Chocolate" Syrup, **56**
Clam Chowder, **94**
Clams Oregano, Baked, **58**
Cocktail Mix, **59**
Coconut Birthday Cake, **112**
Coconut Filling, **112**
Coconut Kisses, **104**
Coconut Orange Custard
   Pie, **116**
Coffee Cake, Orange
   Crumb, **53**
Coffee Cookies, Frosted **106**
Cole Slaw, Sweet 'n Sour, **94**
Confections
   Easy Penuche, **126**
   8-Minute Chocolate
      Fudge, **126**
   Krackle Korn, **125**
   Strawberry Tofu Pop-
      sicles, **125**
**Convenience Food
Substitutes**
   "Chocolate" Syrup, **56**
   Cream-of-Mushroom
      Soup Substitute, **39**
   Fresh Croutons, **44**
   Granola, Homemade, **54**
   Mini-Croutons, **43**
   "Packaged" Bread
      Stuffing, **41**
   Seasoned Bread
      Crumbs, **43**
   Tartar Sauce, **46**
   Tofu "Sour Cream," **40**

Cookies
  Banana Energy Bars, 105
  Breakfast Cookies, 52
  Butterscotch Oatmeal Cookies, 105
  Coconut Kisses, 104
  Filled "Cheese" Cookies, 38
  Frosted Coffee Cookies, 106
  Peanut Butter Scotchies, 106
  Walnut Brownies, 108
Corn Bread, 102
Cranberry Mold, 96
Cranberry Nut Muffins, 52
Croutons, Fresh, 44
Croutons, Mini-, 43

D
Desserts
  Blueberry Tarts, 117
  Butterscotch Swirl Ice Cream, 123
  Cheeseless Cheesecake, 120
  Coconut Orange Custard Pie, 116
  Dream Puffs, 118
  Granola Apple Crisp, 121
  Jewelled Bavarian Cream, 123
  Orange Pineapple Tapioca, 124
  Orange Velvet Sherbet, 122
  Philadelphia Ice Cream, 122
  Pina Colada Tapioca, 124
  Pumpkin Pie, 116
  Rum Mousse, 119
  Strawberry Angel Pie, 117
  Twist O' Lemon, 121
Dieter's Delite Nibblers, 62
Dip, Tangy Vegetable, 62
Dream Puffs, 118

E
Eggnog, Golden, 51

Eggs
  Eggs a la Russe, 59
  Herbed Mushroom Omelet, 79
  Puffed Omelet, 55
  Spanish Omelet, 79
  Spinach Tofu Quiche, 78

F
Fish and Seafood
  Baked Fish Creole, 76
  Creamy Scallop Casserole, 75
  Crunchy Tuna Bake, 75
  Oven Fried Fillets, 74
  Seven Seas Casserole, 74
  Tuna-Tofu Loaf, 77
Frostings and Fillings
  Coconut Filling, 112
  Fluffy Frosting, 113
  Maple Frosting, 109
Fruit Cocktail Cake, 110
Fruit Smoothy, Fresh, 51

G
Golden Sauce, 111
Granola, Homemade, 54
Grapefruit Surprise, 49
Green Beans Lucette, 88

H
Ham-Rice Salad, 97
Hamburger Vegetable Soup, Speedy, 89

K
Krackle Korn, 125

M
Manicotti, Tofu, 76
Maple "Butter", 56
Maple Cake, 108
Maple Cake, Whole Wheat, 114
Maple Frosting, 109

Mayonnaise, Blender, 46
Meat Loaf, Quick Savory, 67
Meat Loaves, Barbecued, 65
Meat Pies, Mini-, 38
Meatballs, Cocktail, 58
Meats
   Barbecued Meat Loaves, 65
   Beef 'n Pepper Steak, 64
   Beef and Vegetable Casserole 66
   Chili Con Carne, 80
   Easy Pot Roast, 65
   Mini-Meat Pies, 38
   Oven Beef Ragout, 66
   Pork Skillet Dinner, 67
   Quick Savory Meatloaf, 67
   Steak and Potato Broil, 63
   Super Easy Pot Roast, 64
Minestrone, 90
Miscellaneous
   Beer Batter, 40
   Cold Cereal, 54
   Maple "Butter", 56
   Squash "Milk", 40
   Tofu "Sour Cream", 40
   Two-way Bread Stuffing, 42
   "Wild" Rice Stuffing, 42
Muffins, Quick Applesauce, 104
Mushroom Omelet, Herbed, 79
Mushroom Soup Substitute, Cream of, 39
Mushrooms, Spicy Marinated, 60

N
Noodle Ring, 84

O
Orange Cake, Moist, 115
Orange-Pineapple Tapioca, 124
Orange Velvet Sherbet, 122

P
Pancakes, 56
Pastry, "Cheese", 37
Peanut Butter Scotchies, 106
Penuche, Easy, 126
Pina Colada Tapioca 124
Pineapple and Carrot Salad, 96
Pineapple-Lime Salad, 96
Pork Chop Skillet Dinner, 67
Pot Roast, Easy, 65
Pot Roast, Super Easy, 64
Potato Casserole, Crunchy, 81
Potatoes, Scalloped, 82
Pound Cake, Coffee Rich, 114
Pumpkin Pie, 116

R
Rice, Barbecue, 83
Rice, Savory Lemon, 83
Rice, Savory Oven-baked, 84
Rum Mousse, 119
Rye Bread, Coffee Can, 100

S
Salad Dressings
   Boiled Salad Dressing, 44
   Fresh Strawberry Dressing, 45
   Italian Dressing, 45
   Plain Dressing, 45
Salads
   Cherry Salad 95
   Cranberry Mold, 96
   Ham-Rice Salad, 97
   Pineapple-Carrot Salad, 96
   Spinach Salad, 98
   Sweet 'n Sour Cole-slaw, 94
Tuna-Macaroni Salad, 97
Sauces
   Golden Sauce, 111
   Tartar Sauce, 46
   White Sauce, 38

Scallop Casserole, Creamy, 75
Scones, 102
Seafood Remoulade, 57
Seven Seas Casserole, 74
Shake, Berry Tasty, 51
"Shake", Creamy, 50

Soups and Stews
Bean Pot Soup, 90
Clam Chower, 94
Cream of Celery Soup, 91
Cream of Mushroom Soup Substitute, 39
Cream of Tomato Soup, 91
Garden Fresh Vegetable Soup, 92
Marie's Bouillabaisse, 93
Minestrone, 90
Speedy Hamburger Soup, 89
Vegetable Bean Soup, 92

Spaghetti, Summertime, 80
Spice Cake, Sarah's, 111
Spinach Pudding, San Antonio, 87
Spinach Salad, 98
Spinach Tofu Quiche, 78
Squash "Milk" 40
Steak and Potato Broil, 63
Strawberry Angel Pie, 117
Strawberry Dressing, Fresh, 45
Strawberry Tofu Popsicles, 125
Stuffing, "Packaged" Bread, 41
Stuffing Two-Way Bread, 42
Stuffing, "Wild" Rice, 42
Sweet Potato Bake, 82

T
Tabooli, 95
Tartar Sauce, 46
Tofu Dip, 61
Tofu Manicotti, 76
Tofu Popsicles, Strawberry, 125
Tofu Quiche, Spinach, 78
Tofu "Sour Cream", 40
Tomato Soup, Cream of, 91
Tomatoes, Savory, 86
Tuna Bake, Crunchy, 75
Tuna-Macaroni Salad, 97
Tuna-Tofu Loaf, 77

V
Vegetable Bean Soup, 92
Vegetable Dip, Tangy, 62
Vegetable Soup, Garden Fresh, 92

Vegetables and Side Dishes
Baked Bean Casserole, 86
Baked Carrots, 87
Barbecue Rice, 83
Crunchy Potato Casserole, 81
Green Beans Lucette, 88
Noodle Ring, 84
San Antonio Spinach Pudding, 87
Savory Lemon Rice, 83
Savory Oven Baked Rice, 84
Savory Tomatoes, 86
Scalloped Potatoes, 82
Sweet Potato Bake, 82
Tabooli, 95
Vegetarian Baked Beans, 85
Zucchini Provencal, 88

W
Wheat Bread, Honey, 99
White Sauce, 38

Better Living Books from Betterway Publications

Please send me the following books:

Quantity	No.	Title	Price	Amount
_____	05-1	**LIVING...WITHOUT MILK,** 3rd ed. (paper)................	$3.95	_____
_____	06-X	**LIVING...WITHOUT MILK,** 3rd ed. (cloth)................	7.95	_____
_____	04-3	**Jackie's BOOK OF HOUSEHOLD CHARTS............**	5.95	_____
		A comprehensive guide to home management and family care. Spiral bound.		
_____	07-8	**Jackie's INDOOR/OUTDOOR GARDENING CHARTS......**	5.95	_____
		A comprehensive gardening guide for the dedicated novice or seasoned gardener. Easy-to-use charts cover all aspects of gardening. Spiral bound.		
_____	03-5	**NUTRI-DIET™ /NUTRI-DIARY™**	3.95	_____
		A practical, nutritionally balanced weight loss and maintenance program. Separate diet guide and diary booklets in an attractive vinyl case.		
		Postage and handling (any quantity)..................		.80
		Total		_____

Please enclose check or money order. Allow four weeks for delivery. Thank you.

Betterway Publications
White Hall, VA 22987

NAME _____

ADDRESS _____

CITY _____ STATE _____ ZIP _____